HOW TO BEAT EXTREME HUNGER

A NEURODIVERSITY-AFFIRMING GUIDE TO FOOD FREEDOM

LIVIA SARA

How to Beat Extreme Hunger © 2024 Livia Sara

All rights reserved. No portion of this book may be reproduced in any form without prior written permission from the publisher or author. Violation of this clause constitutes unlawful piracy and theft of the author's intellectual property.

This book is intended for informational purposes only and does not constitute health or medical advice. The content contained herein is not intended to diagnose, treat, cure, or prevent any condition or disease. Neither the publisher nor the author shall be liable for any damages, including but not limited to special, incidental, consequential, personal, or commercial damages, resulting from use of the information contained in this book. The content reflects the author's research and opinions as of the publication date.

ISBN 979-8-9875398-8-0

eISBN 979-8-9875398-1-1

Book cover by my sister, Mae van Aarsen

For more information, visit www.livlabelfree.com

SAVE YOUR SEAT!

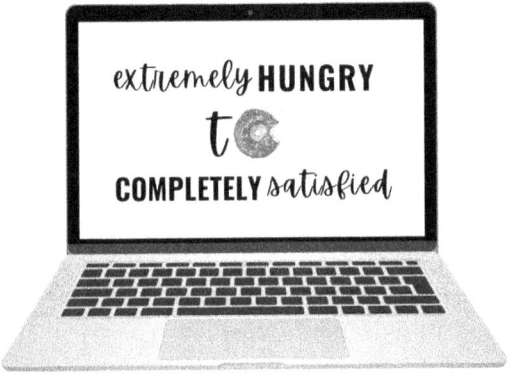

Want to take your healing to the next level? Save your seat in the accompanying course, *Extremely Hungry to Completely Satisfied*, where you'll find visual representations of the concepts in this book, step-by-step guidance, and accountability to help you to overcome extreme hunger: **livlabelfree.com/course**

PRAISE FOR HOW TO BEAT EXTREME HUNGER

"How to Beat Extreme Hunger is an engaging and comprehensive deep dive into understanding a very normal but often misunderstood part of the recovery process. Livia explores this phenomenon from multiple perspectives, helpfully dissecting different types of hunger, the nervous system, hormones, restriction, and much more. Livia is an engaging writer, delving thoroughly into the science of the extreme hunger experience whilst also drawing from her personal journey with deep authenticity and vulnerability. I highly recommend this book to anyone navigating eating disorder recovery!"

— Harriet Frew, The Eating Disorder Therapist

"Liv takes the confusing and often frightening concept of 'extreme hunger' and makes it relatable, logical, and easier to understand. Anyone dealing with extreme hunger from restrictive eating disorders will likely benefit from the way Liv breaks down the what, how, and why of their seemingly out-of-control hunger patterns. With insights ranging from the cognitive, emotional, physical, physiological, and somatic (nervous system), this book is an empathetic and practical guide for getting through this messy part of recovery."

— Stefanie Michele, Binge Eating and Body Image Coach

"In *How to Beat Extreme Hunger*, Livia Sara delivers a refreshing take on overcoming the challenges of extreme hunger with a blend of humor, raw honesty, and genuine understanding. From the very first page, Livia's voice feels like that of a trusted friend who not only acknowledges your struggles but dives deep into the heart of them.

This book is a revelation – a beacon of truth in a sea of misconceptions. Livia fearlessly drops 'truth bombs' that illuminate the hidden aspects of our relationship with food and our bodies. Through her relatable candid storytelling, she unveils the seemingly 'harmless' behaviors that can stop us from overcoming extreme hunger.

Livia doesn't just illuminate the problem; she provides a roadmap out. With a step-by-step approach, she guides readers through the process of claiming true liberation in their relationship with food. Each chapter feels like a breakthrough, with multiple 'ah-ha' moments leading you closer to freedom from the confines of your eating disorder.

What sets *How to Beat Extreme Hunger* apart is Livia's willingness to address topics that most professionals overlook but should know. That's why this book is the key to recovery. Rooted deeply in authenticity, Livia's words serve as a lifeline for those lost in their struggles, resonating deeply with the soul. As you read, you feel deeply heard and understood.

As a food freedom and body love coach, I wholeheartedly believe that *How to Beat Extreme Hunger* is a game-changer for anyone seeking liberation from the grip of extreme hunger. I'll definitely be sending each of my clients a copy! If you're ready to embark on a journey that promises more than overcoming extreme hunger, your search ends here. This book is your guidebook to reclaiming your life and embracing true nourishment, inside and out.

Liv, you're a freaking genius and a positive light in this world!"

— Victoria Kleinsman, Food Freedom & Body Love Coach

"Following in the footsteps of her memoir *Rainbow Girl*, Livia has once again written a truly inspiring and compelling book which I would enthusiastically recommend to anyone in the ED recovery space. As she states in part 1, this book is meant to be a resource, and cannot do the work of recovery for you. Having said that, it is an extremely *powerful* resource and will undoubtedly make taking action easier and less lonesome.

Livia's writing style is truly unique. It's the perfect blend of pertinent scientific facts and bravely written anecdotes from her own lived experience of extreme hunger and ED recovery. Combined, these modalities result in an informative yet compassionate work that will help ease your fears so that you can take the leap into the unknown.

How to Beat Extreme Hunger, in tandem with Livia's impressive online course *Extremely Hungry to Completely Satisfied*, have been integral parts of my recovery journey. I would strongly encourage not only those struggling with an ED but also the therapists, dietitians, and family members involved in the recovery process to take the information eloquently presented here to heart!"

— Valerie, autistic ED warrior and course student

"What a fantastic and incredibly important resource Livia has created in writing the book *How to Beat Extreme Hunger*. It is written in a way that is easy to understand while also including the science behind overcoming extreme hunger. Livia has created a practical guide to navigating what can often be a terrifying part of recovery from a restrictive eating disorder. I wholeheartedly endorse *How to Beat Extreme Hunger* and as an eating disorder recovery coach myself, will definitely be recommending this book to all my clients. Thank you Livia for writing this incredible book!"

— Julia Trehane, Eating Disorder Recovery Coach

"I've read lots of 'recovery' books over the years and I have to say *How to Beat Extreme Hunger* is the best I have ever read! It is so clear, concise, and well researched. Livia's newest book is a must-read for everyone. Not only for those who are in recovery from an eating disorder, but also for those supporting someone in recovery... especially those who are neurodivergent!

For me, finding out that I am neurodivergent while recovering from a restrictive eating disorder (and being in my late 30s!) has been quite the journey. Not only am I learning to navigate life without an eating disorder, but I'm discovering how to embrace being AuDHD and live without restriction. *How to Beat Extreme Hunger* has allowed me to be a lot more compassionate with myself and has helped me view myself and my recovery in a whole new way.

How to Beat Extreme Hunger provides not only science and lived experience, but it clearly explains how integral food is to healing your body, your mind, and your overall outlook on life. Livia goes above and beyond in describing how to rewire your brain, gain a positive relationship with food, and live label free so you can discover true freedom. Please allow Livia to help you on your journey of self discovery and healing!"

— Sabina, autistic ED warrior

"Livia encapsulates a phenomenon experienced by those in eating disorder recovery so incredibly well. The scientific explanations and sheer detail Livia goes into really helped me to understand extreme hunger. It's safe to say I cried a little with relief knowing there's actually a reason for this process and why it's nothing to fear. The wisdom and authenticity Livia expresses in her writing makes you feel as though you are having a deep chat with a friend making it feel all that more personal. This book truly raises awareness to extreme hunger and provides hope for those that feel alone during this experience."

— Shannon, autistic ED warrior

To everyone experiencing extreme hunger and their loved ones. It is a terrifying part of the journey, which is what makes your commitment to healing all the more brave.

CONTENTS

PART 1
MINDSET

1. FEAR	3
2. MOTIVATION	6
3. HABITS	8
4. ACTION	11

PART 2
THE BIOLOGY OF EXTREME HUNGER

5. WHAT IS EXTREME HUNGER?	15
6. WHAT CAUSES EXTREME HUNGER?	18
7. WHEN DOES EXTREME HUNGER HAPPEN?	22

PART 3
UNDERSTANDING HUNGER

8. PHYSICAL HUNGER	29
9. MENTAL HUNGER	32
10. EXERCISE HUNGER	37
11. EATING-INDUCED HUNGER	39
12. EMOTIONAL EATING AND BINGE EATING	41

PART 4
RESTRICTION

13. RESTRICTION AWARENESS	47
14. TYPES OF RESTRICTION	49
15. REWIRING RESTRICTION	58

PART 5
UNRESTRICTED EATING

16. WHAT IS UNRESTRICTED EATING?	61
17. JUNK FOOD	64
18. NIGHT EATING	68
19. BREAKING THE CYCLE	71

PART 6
WEIGHT GAIN

20. TARGET WEIGHTS	75
21. BMI	77
22. WEIGHT RESTORATION AND REDISTRIBUTION	80

PART 7
OTHER BODILY CHANGES

23. THE NERVOUS SYSTEM	87
Central Nervous System	88
Peripheral Nervous System	89
Somatic Nervous System	89
Autonomic Nervous System	89
Polyvagal Theory	90
24. THE ENDOCRINE SYSTEM	95
25. DIGESTIVE ISSUES	98
26. HORMONAL CHANGES	111
Ghrelin	113
Leptin	113
Evolutionary Adaptations to Famine	118
Insulin	122
Metabolism	126
Mood Swings	131
Aches and Pains	132
Edema	133
Puberty, Periods, and PMDD	134
Sleep	153

PART 8
LIVING LABEL FREE

27. TOO MUCH IDENTIFICATION?	165
28. ALL IN RECOVERY	170
29. VICTIMHOOD	174
30. TRIGGERS	178
31. DIET CULTURE	180
32. GUILT	182
33. DISCOVERY	185

What did you think?	187
Also by Livia Sara	189
Endnotes	191
About the Author	199

PART 1

MINDSET

1

FEAR

If you're reading this, it's because you believe it's possible to bEAT extreme hunger. Your mind may be racing with fear, buzzing with questions, and I'm willing to bet there's a voice in your head coming up with a million reasons why your extreme hunger isn't valid. Yet, deep down, you know that a life of fulfillment and satisfaction is possible for you. If you didn't, you wouldn't be here investing the time and energy to achieve that life!

I wrote this book to act as a stepping stone on your journey. I survived an eating disorder, I overcame extreme hunger, and I've had more ups and downs on this messy path called life than I can remember. But I'm now stronger because of it, and I continue to become stronger each day. I've been where you are and come out the other side, which means I know it's 100% possible to overcome extreme hunger and live a life in which you feel satisfied – in every sense of the word. But it wasn't always that way.

When I was experiencing extreme hunger, I feared I would never stop eating, that I would gain weight forever, and that I just had to accept the unlucky fate of being obsessed with food. I believed I had conditioned my body and brain beyond repair. I believed that full recovery from disordered eating was possible for everyone else, but not for me. I believed I was the anomaly for whom recovery wasn't going to work, and therefore I doubted whether it was even worth trying.

Despite my uncertainty, there was always a part of me that knew I had to at least try. And when I say "try," I mean fully commit. Not dip my toes in the possibility of full recovery, not eat a large amount of food only to stop myself after an amount I deemed "acceptable," and not go out to eat only after I had exercised and "deserved" it. When I say I fully committed to recovery, I mean I fully surrendered to the process and everything it would entail.

Yes, I was filled with every fear possible, but what is fear really? Fear is not trusting the outcome. And why didn't I trust the outcome? Because I didn't *know* the outcome. Just as darkness is the absence of light, fear is simply the absence of knowledge. I feared my mental hunger would never go away because I had never provided my brain with evidence that a life without mental hunger was possible. I feared endless weight gain because I'd never given my body the opportunity to eat unrestricted and settle at a healthy weight. I feared I was the "magical unicorn" for whom recovery wasn't possible because I'd never experienced life while being fully recovered.

As ridiculous as they seem to me now, those fears are completely valid. Because it's true: you have zero proof that recovery is going to work for you. There is no guarantee that your mental hunger will ever go away. The outcome of your putting in the work isn't certain. But what *is* certain is that the way you're living right now is making you miserable. The only guarantee you have is that continuing to live this way will continue to make you miserable.

I realized I had nothing to lose and everything to gain, and that is the moment I gathered the confidence to take the leap. As I describe in my memoir *Rainbow Girl*, a massive part of the trust required to take the leap was rooted in the knowledge that I could always go back to my eating disorder. Yep, that's right: if a fully recovered life truly sucks, you can always go back to your eating disorder. But if you continue to engage in your eating disorder without even giving yourself a chance to recover, you'll never be able to buy back the time you missed.

Although it may sound preposterous of me to share the option of returning to your eating disorder at the beginning of a book about overcoming extreme hunger, I'm just being honest. Having this back door open gave me the courage to jump into the unknown. Knowing that I could always go back to what I trusted, to what I knew, gave me the strength I needed to trust what I didn't yet know.

Of course, reaching a place of full recovery made me realize that life is far greater than anything I could have ever imagined, so I'm never going back to my eating disorder. Overcoming my fears by facing them head-on taught me about the acronym for FEAR: FEAR is False Evidence Appearing Real. But when you're stuck in a thought loop convincing you that this evidence isn't actually false, having a back door open can be a powerful motivator. And while we are on the topic of motivation, let's unpack how to stay motivated while bEATing extreme hunger – because you're gonna need it!

2

MOTIVATION

Us humans (and all species) need motivation when we're attempting to do something difficult. Becoming a surgeon, training for a marathon, writing a book…these are all endeavors that require discipline and motivation. When we see someone pursuing such a venture and aspire to do the same, we often ask, "How do you find the motivation?" or "Where do you get the motivation from?" But we are asking the wrong questions. The real question is "*Why* are you motivated?" And the answer has everything to do with the definition of the word "motivation": *a reason or reasons for acting or behaving in a certain way.*

Someone who dedicates their time and energy to becoming a surgeon doesn't do it because they need a job. Their commitment may be fueled by their passion to save lives – their dream of saving lives being their reason to work long hours and say no to other activities. Someone who wakes up early to run several miles a day doesn't do it because they have nothing better to do. Their commitment to increasing their endurance may be driven by their desire to feel the victory of completing a marathon. Someone who writes a book (or several) doesn't do it because they enjoy the eye strain that comes from staring at a computer screen for long hours. Their commitment to getting words onto the page could be fueled by their drive to make an impact and change lives (I'm speaking from personal experience here!).

In all of these cases, the motivation – the reason for acting a certain way – is rooted in a strong *why*. Knowing your why is essential when it comes to overcoming extreme hunger because it gives you a strong enough reason to keep pushing through when the going gets tough. To grasp this concept, it will help to understand how the brain forms and maintains habits.

3

HABITS

I'm sure you've heard the phrase that humans are creatures of habit. That's because we literally are! Every day, you execute tasks without conscious effort. Turning on the shower, brushing your teeth, making your bed – these are all activities you could do practically in your sleep. When you repeat a behavior over and over again, your brain creates a network to store that behavior. This neural network is what we call a habit. Humans' ability to form and maintain habits is the brain's way of increasing its efficiency. If you had to get up every morning and deeply think about how to take a shower, brush your teeth, or make your bed, you'd use up all your precious brainpower before the more important tasks of the day could even begin. Thanks to evolution, these daily activities are mere executions of a behavior you've conditioned your brain to do.

Because your habits – such as the elements of your morning routine – no longer require conscious thought, you have more energy left over for critical thinking and decision-making. Thousands of years ago, such an adaptation would increase your chances of survival, as more energy meant a heightened opportunity to seek out food and protect yourself from danger. This evolutionary adaptation is also why it's so hard to change. If you've repeated a specific behavior over and over again, there must have been a good reason for it. Your brain has come to trust and rely on that behavior and has made it part of its everyday thinking routine. So, when you try to break that routine and do something different, your brain will fight back!

Everyone knows how hard it is to kick a habit. It's why people have such a hard time quitting an addiction, the explanation for terrified partners staying in toxic relationships, and the reason people with eating disorders so badly *want* to recover yet continue to feel overwhelmed by the thought of actually doing so. In the case of an eating disorder (ED), you've conditioned your brain to behave in a certain way after repeatedly giving it reasons to behave in that way. Every time you see a cookie and eat an apple instead, you're conditioning your brain that you are someone who doesn't eat cookies. When you've repeated this behavior enough times, your brain no longer even has to think about whether you're going to choose the cookie or the apple; grabbing the apple becomes the default. By always choosing the apple, you've given your brain reason to believe it should create a neural network that supports eating only apples. Why would it create a neural network for cookies if you'd never use that network anyways? That would be a total waste of energy. And the brain doesn't mess around when it comes to efficiency.

Your brain's ability to form and maintain habits circles directly back to fear, which, as you learned in chapter 1, comes down to lacking knowledge of a certain outcome. The reason you fear taking the action steps necessary to reach full recovery – eating the cookie, buying bigger clothes, resting – is because your brain doesn't already have neural networks that support these actions. Because it lacks these neural networks, it also lacks the knowledge of what would happen if you took those actions…and because it lacks the knowledge, it doesn't trust the outcome of taking those actions.

So what happens when you commit to full recovery and you finally take those actions? Your brain has to work overtime to form new neural pathways. This formation costs additional energy, which is why recovery from an eating disorder is so damn exhausting. In essence, recovery comes down to dismantling old neural networks and creating new ones. You're weakening your "old brain" while simultaneously building a new one. Although this may sound discouraging considering the brain's aversion to change, the concept's manifestation is actually quite promising. If a habit is simply the formation of a neural network and your eating disorder is a combination of neural networks, becoming free from an eating disorder boils down to creating new habits. Of course, creating new habits isn't easy, but you know what they say: "It isn't going to be easy, but it's going to be worth it." Cliché, I know, but there's a reason such phrases are clichés – because they're true.

4

ACTION

Recovery from an eating disorder is like working with a row of dominoes. Similar to how knocking down the initial domino causes the succeeding dominoes to fall without further interference, taking recovery-oriented actions makes it easier to take more recovery-oriented actions down the line. Tackling that first domino – your first fear food, your first rest day, your first extreme hunger feast – is the hardest, but once the dominoes start falling, you become unstoppable!

I know what you're thinking: "It's the very idea of my hunger being unstoppable that I'm so afraid of!" And that's exactly why I wrote this book. Now that you understand the mechanisms behind fear, motivation, and habits, it's time to give your brain the knowledge it needs to trust your extreme hunger journey.

In the following chapters, I'll tell you everything there is to know about extreme hunger: why it happens, when it happens, who it happens to, what to expect when you honor it, and how to build a life in which you feel satisfied and free. The information in this book is a combination of scientific research and lived experience, both from my personal journey with extreme hunger and from the hundreds of clients I've guided to freedom. I promise to hold nothing back. This book, along with my course *Extremely Hungry to Completely Satisfied*, is the resource pair I wish I had when I was going through this terrifying part of recovery. It is therefore my greatest honor to have created it for you.

Please keep in mind that this book is merely that – a resource. It provides you with information and insight to inspire you to do the work, but it cannot do the work for you. Only you can take the action steps necessary to create new neural networks in your brain. Only you can supply your brain with the knowledge it needs to trust the outcome. Only you can prove to your brain that your "fears" are False Evidence Appearing Real.

This book contains tips and questions to ask yourself, and further action steps can be found in the accompanying course, *Extremely Hungry to Completely Satisfied*. Not only does the course provide a visual representation of the concepts laid out in this book, but it lays the groundwork for taking action and offers an added layer of accountability. While this book can be read by anyone and everyone all by their lonesome, I created my course so that you don't have to go through this process in solitude.

As Katie, one of my past course students, so eloquently remarked, "I felt like I had someone walking beside me, guiding me through while I was taking her course." Katie went through my course before I wrote this book, and perhaps you are reading this book without having gone through my course. Both resources are wonderful on their own, but just as you need two dominoes for them to have a domino effect, the book and the course together create an unstoppable resource. To maximize your healing potential and enroll in *Extremely Hungry to Completely Satisfied*, visit the course page on my website: livlabelfree.com/course. Now, let's bEAT extreme hunger!

PART 2

THE BIOLOGY OF EXTREME HUNGER

5

WHAT IS EXTREME HUNGER?

Let's start with the basics, shall we? There is obviously no dictionary definition of the term "extreme hunger," but there are definitions of the words "hunger" and "extreme." According to Merriam-Webster Dictionary, these terms can be defined as follows:

Hunger: a craving or urgent need for food or a specific nutrient.

Extreme: reaching a high or the highest degree, i.e., very great.

When we put these two terms together, the resulting definition of extreme hunger is *a very urgent need for food or specific nutrients.*

Notice that this definition does not specify one type of hunger. This is a crucial point to be aware of, as a common misconception when experiencing extreme hunger is that the hunger is only "valid" when it is purely physical. This belief acts as an enormous hindrance to reaching full recovery because it often leads to the denial or invalidation of alternative types of hunger that are just as valid as physical hunger (more on this in part 3).

Throughout this book, I invite you to shift your perspective on certain labels, as I believe labels are at the root of limitations. The only reason you fear eating more is because you've labeled the act of eating more as "bad" and "wrong." You've conditioned your brain to believe this, making it a belief you currently trust. In the same vein, you may believe you are "not sick enough" to be experiencing extreme hunger because you're already "weight restored" or "didn't restrict for long enough." But all these stipulations – valid, sick enough, weight restored, duration of restriction – are labels. You will learn more about setting yourself free from labels in part 8, but for now, let's debunk the label that appears in the very title of this book: "extreme."

In my work as an eating disorder recovery coach, I often hear the phrase "my hunger is *too* extreme." This belief stems from the brain's frame of reference, which has attached labels and limitations to food. Someone may compare their desire for food and specific nutrients not only to the intake of those around them but also to what their current frame of reference has labeled "normal" and "appropriate." But because an eating disorder distorts your frame of reference, you must be open to alternative views in order to create new and healthy neural networks. An alternative to the view that your hunger is "too extreme" is the perspective that it isn't your hunger that's extreme – all the restriction and compensation leading up to it are!

That being said, you may ask, "Well, if it's not actually the hunger that's extreme, why use the term *extreme* hunger at all?" My honest answer is for the sake of semantics. In the end, the way we use words and communicate with each other is all through labels. In part 8, we'll go deeper into labels and how I advise "living label free," but for now, just consider that labels are inevitable and that there are two types of labels: limiting labels and functional labels. What defines a limiting label from a functional one has to do with the intention behind the label. Labeling food as "bad" doesn't help you function better – it sets you up for restriction, as intending to restrict actually is the intention behind the label. In contrast, labeling a book with the term "extreme hunger" in the title helps reach the people the book aims to help – you! I use the term "extreme hunger" throughout this book, as well as in my other content on this topic, because it serves an important function: reaching and helping people who are currently experiencing a terrifying and often lonely part of recovery. If we all had some kind of sixth sense that attracted us to the resources and understanding we needed without using potentially misleading words or phrases, I definitely wouldn't be preceding the word "hunger" with "extreme." Because your hunger isn't extreme. You just need a lot of food, and there's a reason for that!

6

WHAT CAUSES EXTREME HUNGER?

In the previous chapter, we established that your hunger isn't extreme – the restriction and compensation leading up to it is. Your heightened hunger is your body's way of making up for all that restriction and compensation to get you healthy again. In fact, there's even a scientific term for this biological response: post-starvation hyperphagia. It is defined as *an increase in the sensation of hunger and overeating after a period of chronic energy deprivation that can be part of an autoregulatory phenomenon attempting to restore body weight.*[1]

The increased hunger and overeating are nothing more than the body's reactions to chronic energy deprivation. But how did you get into chronic energy deprivation in the first place? We can break down this biological concept by understanding the terms "energy deficit" and "energy debt."

Energy deficit occurs when you consume an inadequate amount of food to meet your body's unique nutritional needs. A healthy body is in energy balance, meaning it's receiving the same amount of calories that it is putting out, i.e., "burning." The reason you may feel hungrier after a workout or a long exam is because your body demands additional energy – and it is trying to bring you back into balance by requesting additional food.

You go into energy deficit when the amount of calories you are taking in is insufficient to support the proper functioning of your body. The most common causes of energy deficit are dieting, overexercise, chronic illness, and stress. All of these circumstances deplete the body of the energy it needs to ensure healthy functioning.

When your brain learns that your body is in energy deficit, your brain has reason to believe you are in a famine environment. More specifically, it's your brain stem that believes you are in a famine environment. Why else wouldn't you be consuming enough food? The brain stem is the oldest part of your evolved brain and has the sole role of ensuring your survival. The brain stem is the first part of the brain to develop, and because some animals, such as reptiles, have only a brain stem, it is often referred to as the primal brain or the reptilian brain.

The reptilian brain is responsible for regulating autonomic functions, including breathing and heart rate, but it also plays a role in the fight-or-flight response. Because its sole purpose is to ensure your survival, the brain stem does not think – it acts. If someone poured boiling water on your hand, you would automatically pull away without thinking. That immediate response is your brain stem in action! Your brain stem does not consult with the logical parts of your brain; in dangerous situations, there is simply no time to think about what the "logical" course of action would be.

A lack of adequate resources is one of the biggest threats to human survival. So, when you are in energy deficit, your brain stem perceives a threat. Because your brain stem acts on impulse, it doesn't matter if you know *logically* that you're not in a famine environment – all your brain stem perceives is a lack of adequate resources.

When your brain believes that resources are scarce, it causes the body to start economizing. Your body will become very selective about where it allocates energy. If your body continued to burn just as much energy as if you were healthy and resource-rich, you'd run out of energy fairly quickly…which would result in death. And that's exactly what your primal brain is primed to prevent! In an effort to conserve energy, your body will slow down bodily processes, including your heart rate, digestion, and metabolism. You will also feel cold as your body tries to release the minimum amount of heat (energy) possible.

For a while, your body may be able to sustain this energy conservation, as the human body is an excellent adapter. There are times when resources simply do become scarce – otherwise, animals would never migrate or hibernate. Thanks to evolution, your body is equipped with the impulses it needs to seek out food and survive. Because your body trusts these instincts, a temporary period of hunger is no serious threat. Think about having to wait for a while at a restaurant. You know – and therefore trust – that dinner will be served soon, so you stay seated instead of going to another restaurant. The situation would only become threatening if your meal never arrived and you also skipped dessert, barely ate breakfast, and continued undereating (and perhaps simultaneously overexercising). Over time, your energy deficit turns into *a period of chronic energy deprivation* (remember the definition of post-starvation hyperphagia?) and you start building up energy debt.

Because your body has no idea when food will be readily available again, it slows down more and will even stop nonessential life processes. One of the most common examples is a missing period in people who menstruate – why would your body waste energy on menstruation if it needed to use that precious energy to keep your heart beating? Not to mention, how is your body supposed to trust you to feed a baby when it can't trust you to feed yourself?

Despite your body's signals of deprivation, you continue your day-to-day life and continue to use your limited energy for other activities, whether that's strenuous exercise or attending work or school. If your body has no energetic reserves to support these activities, it's going to seek places within the body to get that energy. Your body will literally start eating itself up, leaching energy from your organs, bones, and other biological processes. The buildup of energy debt can lead to serious long-term health consequences such as organ failure, osteoporosis, and permanent brain damage. This is all very scary, which is why it's time to stop waiting until you finally feel "ready" to recover.

Now – before you think "Oh, it's probably too late anyways, I've already messed my body up!" – allow me to share a powerful quote with you: *The best time to plant a tree was ten years ago. The second-best time is today.* As I mentioned before, the body is an excellent adapter and *will* heal when given the resources to do so.

Before I fully committed to recovery, I believed it was too late. I developed an eating disorder when I was eleven years old and didn't have my first period until I was almost nineteen. I was even told by health professionals that I would never be able to bear children. I was told I would just have to "manage" an eating disorder for the rest of my life. But was I really going to spend the rest of my life according to someone else's poor prediction of it? I'd already spent enough years at the mercy of my illness. By committing to full recovery, I proved every professional wrong and in turn, my body proved to me how capable it was of healing.

Perhaps now you decide you're done living life on someone else's watch and you commit to full recovery for yourself. You start eating more, stop exercising, gain some weight…and BOOM! All the dominoes start to topple and you cannot stop thinking about food. Your (mental) hunger becomes an invisible force that won't stop tugging at you until you've raided the kitchen and eaten everything in sight with so much urgency. And before you know it, you're lying on the couch in the fetal position, unable to move because you're so full. The only way I'm able to describe this experience with such accuracy is because I've been there – many times.

7

WHEN DOES EXTREME HUNGER HAPPEN?

When I first came into contact with extreme hunger, I thought my body was broken. I had been deemed "weight restored" and had already gotten my first period. I believed I wasn't "supposed" to gain more weight at that point. Yet there I was, overtaken by an insatiable desire for all the nut butter, cookies, pastries, cakes, ice cream, and sugary cereals my tummy could hold. Had I conditioned my body and brain to become addicted to food in the process of learning how to eat again? Was I now "swinging to the other side" and developing binge-eating disorder?

In an effort to prevent my worst nightmare from becoming a reality, I created safety mechanisms around my intake. I would read or take a nap to distract myself from the hunger. I would load up on vegetables and high-volume foods to physically satiate myself. I would avoid my favorite aisles at the grocery store so I wouldn't be tempted to grab another five boxes of cookies. But all these attempts to control myself and to keep my hunger at bay made my hunger all the more extreme. It wasn't until I stopped hiding from my hunger – until I stopped clinging to restriction and gave myself permission to swing to the side of nonstop eating – that I eventually stopped swinging. To understand why this approach works, let's take a little physics lesson.

I'm sure you've heard of Sir Isaac Newton before, as he is one of the most influential figures in the history of science. Did you know our physics friend was most likely autistic, too? Thanks to his genius mind, we are able to understand most of what we know about energy and motion using Newton's three laws of motion. When it comes to understanding the root cause of extreme hunger, Newton's third law is especially useful. It states *for every action, there is an equal and opposite reaction*. Your extreme hunger is simply an equal and opposite reaction to all the energy deficit and debt you've been building up. To visualize this concept, we can use Newton's Cradle. The further the outermost ball on the left swings (energy deficit), the further the outermost ball on the right will swing in the opposite direction (extreme hunger). This "hunger cradle," as well as a visual representation of everything described in this book, can be found in the accompanying course *Extremely Hungry to Completely Satisfied* (livlabelfree.com/course). Bringing this concept back to biology, the extreme hunger "ball" on the right can only start to move when the ball on the left aligns with the other balls, i.e., when you are already on your way toward coming out of chronic energy deficit.

When I encountered extreme hunger, I didn't understand why it was happening after I'd already gained so much weight. *Shouldn't I have been hungrier when I was eating less, not more?* Given our earlier discussion of energy conservation and the understanding of our reptilian brain, it is completely logical to experience extreme hunger at a later stage of recovery, when you have already gained weight and moved away from that energy deficit.

As mentioned in the previous chapter, your body will be very selective in expending energy when you are in energy deficit. Lack of incoming energy signals a famine to your brain stem, which adapts to its perceived environment. Every action in the body requires fuel, from a single heartbeat to a rumbling stomach. So, when your body isn't receiving enough fuel, certain actions will slow down or cease. Your heart beats with a decreased frequency, and physical hunger cues may dissipate entirely. Because your body no longer trusts that a physical hunger cue will result in the consumption of food, it will use that energy for other biological actions.

Even though you may not have physical hunger cues while in energy deficit and therefore may not *feel* hungry, it doesn't mean you *aren't* hungry. Because what was the definition of hunger again? *A craving or urgent need for food or a specific nutrient.* Whether you are in energy deficit or not, all humans experience cravings and an urgent need for food and nutrients. When you think of hunger, you may immediately think of a growling stomach. Sure, a growling stomach can be an indication of hunger, but it is merely one of many signs. Feeling tired, dizzy, lightheaded, or weak are all physical signs that the body is in urgent need of nutrients – and we haven't even gotten to the mental signs! You will learn all about other types of hunger and how to recognize them in the next section of this book, but for now, let's come back to the question of why extreme hunger occurs later in recovery.

When you start eating more and gaining weight, you are signaling to your brain that it is in fact not in a famine environment. Yay! Equipped with the knowledge that you have resources at your disposal, your brain stem now trusts that you will make use of those resources – that's what the body is primed to do. Because you have been in energy deficit for a prolonged period of time and also have a hefty amount of energy debt to pay off, you require a significant amount of food. Not only do you require a particular amount of energy to support you on a daily basis (to meet your unique metabolic baseline needs), but you also require the energy necessary to repair all the damage done during the time you were building up energy debt.

This incredible energy requirement is what triggers your brain stem to act impulsively around food. It causes you to eat with a sense of urgency because your brain stem has no idea how long this abundance is going to last. After all the time you spent acting as if resources were scarce, how is your brain stem to know there's not another famine right around the corner?

During my own period of extreme hunger, I was afraid of eating even just one cookie or one spoonful of nut butter. I feared that as soon as I started, I wouldn't be able to stop until everything was gone. I remember feeling so out of control as I shoved endless slices of cake down my throat, barely even tasting what I was eating. No matter how many times I told myself to "eat mindfully," it was as if some invisible force took over. It turns out, that invisible force was my survival instinct.

I also remember wanting to shortcut my way to intuitive eating. I thought as long as I ate "balanced" and "healthy" meals with a sweet treat thrown in here and there, I could have the "food freedom" so many people on the internet promote. I thought I didn't need to consume the large amounts of high-calorie foods my body was craving because "normal people don't do that." But trying to go from a place of restriction and deprivation directly to your unique version of food freedom without it looking messy in the process is like asking a toddler to become an adult without allowing them to first be a teenager. Plus, what does "normal" even mean? If you've learned anything from this book so far, you know that "normal" is just another restrictive label.

As the saying goes, change happens outside of your comfort zone. This is because the brain learns through gaining knowledge, which it does through the actions you take. The first time you take a new course of action, it will be uncomfortable – but that's only because it's unfamiliar. For so long, you've abided by your eating disorder's rules and beliefs, and now it's time to write your own code of conduct. To provide your brain and body with the knowledge that your new (and true) beliefs can be trusted, you must take actions aligned with those beliefs. The brain will observe and learn that these beliefs lead to a much better life!

Your brain stem plays a vital role in this process, as its impulsive, survivalist nature prompts you to feel a great and urgent need for food to get you out of energy deficit, pay back the built-up energy debt, and bring you back to a place in which you are happy and healthy. When going through extreme hunger, you will be consuming more calories than you are putting out – so no, it will not work for you to just eat a "normal amount" of food. The only way for your body to trust you again – the only way for your brain stem to learn that resources are not scarce – is to provide your body and brain with proof that resources are truly abundant. Providing yourself with that proof starts with giving yourself permission – permission to eat, to heal, and to trust your body's instincts.

PART 3

UNDERSTANDING HUNGER

In the previous section, you learned the science behind extreme hunger: what causes it, why it happens, and when it happens. I don't think I need to tell you that the experience can be absolutely terrifying. Otherwise, you wouldn't be reading this book! But what did we learn about fear in the first chapter? Fear is a lack of trust, and a lack of trust is a lack of knowledge.

In the following chapters, I will be explaining the different ways in which (extreme) hunger may present itself. Gaining knowledge of these different ways was a crucial part of my own journey to bEATing extreme hunger because it allowed me to honor each type of hunger without judgment.

Before I understood the four types of hunger I'm about to share, I believed that my desire to continue eating past physical fullness was emotional eating. I believed that eating to the point where I felt like I was going to explode – yet still wanted to keep eating – made me a binge eater. In fact, I was even told to "be careful not to eat too much" by a healthcare professional! Whether you are experiencing these same fears, have been given the same "warning," or just want to become more in tune with your body and its cues, stay tuned!

8

PHYSICAL HUNGER

Physical hunger is the type of hunger most people associate with the idea of feeling hungry. It can be indicated by a rumbling stomach, as mentioned previously, but fatigue, lethargy, dizziness, or irritability can all be signs of physical hunger as well. Referring back to our definition of hunger from chapter 5, physical hunger can be interpreted as *any physical sign or symptom that implies a craving or desire for food or specific nutrients.* In the case of extreme hunger, feelings of physical hunger are often described as possessing a "bottomless pit hunger."

While many individuals in recovery from restrictive eating or overexercise will experience this seemingly insatiable physical hunger, you may never experience extreme hunger in the physical sense – and that's okay! It doesn't make your hunger any less valid or real. As an autistic individual, I know firsthand what it's like to have unreliable physical hunger cues. I believe that this very fact was a massive contributor to the development of my eating disorder. As I think back to when my eating disorder started, I remember not feeling hungry. And in nutrition class at school during that time, I was told you shouldn't eat when you're not hungry, which my literal mind took a little too close to heart.

My difficulty recognizing physical cues – and sometimes total inability to do so – has to do with interoception, or rather, the lack of it. Interoception, also known as the eighth sense, helps you monitor the inner state of your body. It helps you regulate your emotions and understand whether you're hungry, thirsty, in pain, too hot, or too cold. Your interoceptive awareness – along with other mechanisms in the body – plays a big role in maintaining bodily homeostasis. Although the word "balance" may immediately come to mind when thinking of homeostasis, it's important to recognize that homeostasis as a construct was never meant to reflect a static state. The term was originally coined by Walter Cannon, who stated, "The coordinated physiological reactions which maintain most of the steady states in the body are so complex, and so peculiar to the living organism, that it has been suggested that a specific designation for these states be employed—homeostasis."[1] Cannon's definition of homeostasis encompasses the dynamic feedback and regulation processes necessary for a living organism to maintain internal states within a functional range. Unfortunately, the term "homeostasis" has lost its true meaning in the popular imagination and is frequently used synonymously with "balance," representing a static internal level.

If you are at all familiar with the language used on social media around eating and living healthfully, you know the term "balance" is not used sparingly: "What I eat in a day to stay *balanced*." "How I *balanced* my blood sugar." "Clean eating to *balance* your hormones." Although these clickbaity titles may provide a sense of having found the answer to your perceived problems, the very endeavor of achieving balance is a problem in and of itself. Clinically, stasis in the body is a sign of severe physiologic compromise. Just think about it: the only time a heart rate monitor is completely balanced is when it's a flat line. The only time your digestion is balanced is when nothing is moving. Change is synonymous to life, meaning stagnation aligns with a lack of life. And isn't living the very thing you're after?

I didn't realize my pining for balance was utopian until it nearly killed me. In the depths of my eating disorder, I always wanted everything to be the same. That way, I could safeguard myself against analysis paralysis, which I believe is an adaptive mechanism for individuals who lack interoceptive awareness. When you don't think you can trust your inner cues to tell you what you want to eat, you revert to external rules. You believe food needs to be "perfect" in order to be "worth it," which results in overthinking your food and movement decisions. But because there is no "perfect" way to eat or move – or heck, *live* – we become "paralyzed" by our ongoing mental analyses. In turn, this ongoing state of nervous contemplation leads to heightened anxiety, yet another concept that can be better understood through an interoceptive lens.

Our emotional experience is coordinated by interoceptive awareness, meaning lack of interoception can lead to difficulty recognizing and expressing emotions. This trait is known as alexithymia. Someone with alexithymia may be overresponsive to inner cues of fear or worry, resulting in those increased feelings of anxiety. When you are in an ongoing state of anxiety, your brain constantly believes you are in a threatening situation and thus puts physical hunger cues on the back burner. This state of anxiety can contribute to the digestive issues commonly experienced during healing from disordered eating, which also results from your body needing to build up its tolerance for (increased amounts of) food. Because the recovery process itself can already feel so threatening (think back to chapter 3 and the discussion about how the brain is fearful of new situations), it is not uncommon to experience heightened anxiety and, therefore, experience even more confusion around physical hunger cues. If you resonate, you'll want to pay extra close attention to the following chapters on mental hunger. Extreme hunger does not discriminate, and it will find other ways to inform you of its presence if it's unable to do so physically.

9

MENTAL HUNGER

Mental hunger, as the name suggests, is *any mental sign of your desire or need for food and/or specific nutrients.* Unlike physical hunger, mental hunger can be a lot harder to recognize. Not only are the signs more subtle, but you have been conditioned – by diet culture and by your eating disorder – to believe mental hunger cannot be trusted.

To better understand the nuanced nature of your beliefs around mental hunger and other food-related judgments, it can be helpful to define diet culture. As I use the term, diet culture can be summed up as the collective set of social expectations that prioritize and glorify thinness through the promotion of restrictive eating habits. Diet culture involves the societal pressure to conform to idealistic (and often unrealistic) beauty standards, spreading the pervasive belief that appearance and body shape are more important than overall health. Similar to how our society is so built on patriarchy that gender biases often go unnoticed, diet culture is so ingrained that you are likely unaware of its influence on you. One of the most prominent illustrations of diet culture's infiltration brings me to a specific exchange I had with my therapist when I was going through extreme hunger.

When I told my therapist about my first "binge" (I hesitate to use that word because honoring hunger isn't bingeing, but that's how I saw it at the time), she told me, "Sometimes, when we can no longer use our restrictive behaviors to cope with our emotions, we will turn to food." My therapist went on to inform me that my strong desire to eat lots of food was a way for me to "numb my emotions" and "fill an emotional void," a void that my eating disorder had apparently filled previously. After hearing this horrific information, I turned to Dr. Google to research my "symptoms," which included eating large amounts of food past physical fullness, eating rapidly, feeling out of control around food, and feeling guilty or ashamed afterward. Countless search results led me to the same conclusion: I was developing binge-eating disorder.

In an effort to protect myself from "swinging to the other side," I implemented every "hack" I had learned on my disordered eating journey: I ate high-volume foods, used smaller plates and bowls to visually make my food look like more, took small bites, avoided having anything "unhealthy" in the house, and wouldn't allow myself to eat before or after certain times. I justified all of this restriction by reminding myself I was "weight restored" and it would simply take time for my body to realize it no longer needed all that food to gain weight.

However, the more I clung to the rituals and routines that had kept me stuck in my eating disorder in the first place, the stronger my desire for food became. I was thinking, planning, and dreaming about food 24/7. I feared having any open blocks of time or even going to bed because the lack of distraction would open the gateway to intensified food fantasies: eating entire cakes I would never make, spreading butter on toast I would never eat, and licking my fingers over chocolate bars I would never buy. This constant obsession with food and everything that has to do with food (including thoughts that you need to exercise to "deserve" food) is the definition of mental hunger, my friend.

As I stated earlier, the reason you believe your mental hunger cannot be trusted is because you have been conditioned to believe this. Due to diet culture's idealization of weight and appearance over true mental and physical health, you (and other members of society) receive the message that any behaviors contradictory to the pursuit of thinness should be avoided at all costs. Even when these behaviors are necessary for survival – such as eating enough food for your unique needs – you are bombarded with warnings that your own biological cues cannot be trusted. You are sold the promise that weight loss will solve all your problems. But where did this toxicity even come from? Why is diet culture so prominent in the first place?

The harsh reality is that we live in a fatphobic society in which looking "healthy" on the outside shields the type of health that really matters: how your body is functioning internally. But because inner health – including state of mind and the functioning of physical systems – cannot be measured with arbitrary numbers such as body mass index (BMI) or clothing size, you are judged and labeled based on external representations. For example, if someone is battling an eating disorder while presenting with a BMI that falls within "normal" range, their experience is often invalidated by professionals. Similarly, someone who is deemed "weight restored" may be told their extreme hunger is actually emotional eating. Not only can such comments impose feelings of guilt and shame, but they can act as a barrier to internalizing the empowerment that supports the action steps necessary to reach full recovery. Thankfully, your body is a smart cookie. It doesn't listen to bullshit advice and instead activates biological blueprints, including the implementation of mental hunger. Now that you know how the body adapts to perceived famine, we can unpack the (very vital) role mental hunger plays in getting you back to your unique state of nourishment.

Whether you are in chronic energy deficit or are well on your way to coming out of it, anyone and everyone with a history of restriction will experience mental hunger. I know that's a bold statement to make, but if you're alive, it means you have a brain stem. And if you have a brain stem, it means you have survival instincts that will prompt you to seek out food. When your body doesn't (yet) trust that resources are abundant, it will continue to conserve energy until you prove that it's safe to expend energy. Because physical hunger cues are a costly investment from an energy perspective, the body is not yet willing to sacrifice its precious energy on sending them out. Every time the body sent them out and you didn't respond, you were conditioning your brain to believe that spending energy on physical hunger cues was a "waste of energy." And the body does not waste energy! On top of that, if you lack interoceptive awareness and don't respond to physical hunger cues because you are unable to recognize them rather than out of purposeful restriction, you are also (consciously or unconsciously) conditioning your brain to think that physical hunger cues aren't "worth it."

Equipped with the knowledge that physical hunger cues are not the best way to expend energy, your brain will create alternative ways to acquire calories. And what is the most cost-effective way to signal you to seek out food? To think about food! Sending a thought costs way less energy than sending a physical cue. Mental hunger is the form in which extreme hunger is present even in people who are in chronic energy deficit because it signals hunger while conserving the maximum amount of energy. I never fail to marvel at the magic of the human body.

So how do you recognize mental hunger? Deep down, I'm sure you already know. If you're thinking about food – whether this is scrolling through food porn on social media, watching "What I Eat in a Day" videos, planning meals and recipes, fantasizing about food, or calculating what you need to do to deserve more food – you are mentally hungry. You've likely known this for a long time but haven't given yourself permission to honor the mental hunger due to your underlying fears. You may have fears that you will never stop eating, that you've trained your brain to be obsessed with food, that you'll "swing to the other side" or become "emotionally attached" to food if you eat when you're mentally (i.e., not physically) hungry…but remember that FEAR is nothing more than False Evidence Appearing Real. You have no knowledge of what will happen if you honor your mental hunger, and that's why your brain doesn't trust it. So give your brain a reason to trust mental hunger; equip your brain with the knowledge it needs to perceive abundance.

Aside from thinking about food and everything that has to do with food, there are two other forms of hunger that deserve their own discussion: exercise hunger and eating-induced hunger.

10

EXERCISE HUNGER

Exercise hunger is a form of mental hunger. And before you think "Oh! Well, if thinking about food means I need to eat food, then thinking about exercise means I need to exercise," not so fast. In fact, if your behaviors around food and exercise depend on each other, you are most likely experiencing the exercise form of mental hunger. This is because you are trying to work out (no pun intended) ways in which you can eat more food. When I was still in the grip of my disordered relationship with food and exercise, I would obsessively plan my workouts and force myself to move, even when I was tired and didn't feel like it. Meal and snack times were the highlights of my life, so I would do anything I could to keep them the same – even if that meant pushing through exhaustion.

When you understand the purpose of mental hunger – to prompt food-seeking behavior in the most energy-efficient way possible – thinking about exercise in order to deserve food falls logically into the same category. Although exercise hunger isn't as obvious as the mental hunger described in the previous chapter, it is just as significant and necessary to honor.

So how do you recognize exercise hunger? If you are thinking about exercise and feel you need to eat differently if you don't do said exercise, you are experiencing exercise hunger. You must honor it in the exact same way as any other type of hunger because it indicates your need for nutrients. Keep in mind that thinking about exercise is thinking about any form of movement or compensation: walking, pacing, doing chores, unnecessary shopping, taking the stairs instead of the elevator, not allowing yourself to sit down, etc. Engaging in any behavior that aims to negate a number of calories consumed is a sign that you are experiencing exercise hunger and must eat more.

11

EATING-INDUCED HUNGER

The fourth type of hunger worth noting is eating-induced hunger, or hunger that has been triggered by eating. I first became aware of this type of hunger when I was in recovery from my eating disorder, but I quickly learned that it's something I've experienced my whole life. I could never understand why I rarely felt physically hungry before I started eating, only to become ravenous halfway through or right after a meal. When I discovered at the age of twenty that I am autistic and simultaneously started learning about interoception, this type of hunger began to make more sense to me.

From a biological perspective, the body's ability to sense physical hunger during or after caloric consumption is quite logical. As discussed in chapter 8, physical hunger cues will not be sent out if the brain does not trust you will respond to them. This absence of response can be due to a lack of interoceptive awareness but also may result from being in energy deficit. Whatever the reason, eating-induced hunger stems from a lack of trust.

In the case of interoception, there is no trust in your body's communicative abilities, including the recognition of hunger when you need to eat. In the case of energy deficit, your brain lacks confidence in the environment's ability to supply food, which mutes physical hunger cues to conserve energy. Whether interoceptive difficulties and energy deficit present simultaneously or disparately, both convey scarcity, which your body translates to danger. When you start eating, however, your brain learns that resources are not at all scarce, and it is therefore allowed to initiate the digestive process, triggering those hunger cues.

Eating-induced hunger can be incredibly scary because of its unpredictability. Even today, I often find myself making a meal only to realize I am much hungrier and will eat loads more after! But remember, unpredictability isn't a bad thing. Nothing in life is 100% guaranteed. The only guarantee you have is that you'll continue to have extreme (mental) hunger if you don't honor all types of hunger right now – including eating-induced hunger.

12

EMOTIONAL EATING AND BINGE EATING

I've mentioned the terms "emotional eating" and "binge eating" a few times because I personally worried a lot about these concepts when I experienced extreme hunger. And I know I'm not the only one, as I receive messages almost daily about these topics. Because many of the behaviors exhibited during extreme hunger match the diagnostic criteria for binge-eating disorder (BED), individuals coming out of energy deficit often fear they are "swinging to the other side," or overcorrecting after restrictive eating patterns. What's worse is that I know I'm also not the only one who's been told by professionals that my symptoms were a sign that I was developing emotional-eating or binge-eating tendencies.

These ideas and statements are incredibly dangerous because they are coming from a standpoint that lacks comprehension of both extreme hunger and BED. As explained thus far, the root cause of extreme hunger is restriction. When you do not consume a sufficient number of calories for your unique energetic needs, your body goes into energy deficit and your brain perceives a food shortage. This perceived scarcity triggers your primal brain to focus on food, as food is necessary for survival. When you start eating adequately and prove to your brain that resources are plentiful, you are giving your body the golden ticket to heal.

Healing requires additional energy, and thus your eating behaviors will naturally reflect those of binge-eating disorder: eating large amounts of food, eating rapidly, and feeling guilty after eating (because you've conditioned your brain that eating more food is "wrong"). I guide you through the full criteria of binge-eating disorder in Module 5 of *Extremely Hungry to Completely Satisfied*, but the fifth criterion of BED is the most relevant in separating it from extreme hunger: *The binge eating is not associated with the regular use of inappropriate compensatory behavior (e.g., purging, fasting, excessive exercise) and does not occur exclusively during the course of anorexia nervosa or bulimia nervosa.*[1]

In other words, criterion 5 states that if there is *any* form of restriction or compensation involved before or after the binge eating occurs, the behavior does not qualify as binge-eating disorder. To elaborate, someone who has diagnosable BED does not need to come out of energy deficit like you do. I know what you may be thinking now: "But what if I'm out of energy deficit and I keep experiencing urges to binge?" To this, my answer is: How is this belief holding you back from living a better life?

Continuing to restrict and suppress your extreme hunger now is allowing fear to rule your life. Engaging in "what if X goes wrong" thoughts keeps you in a constant state of anxiety and will never bring you closer to a life that's free from the torturous food and movement obsessions. As you learned in part 1 of this book, you only fear something because your brain doesn't know something. Thus, the only way to know if you'll ever stop eating and feel satisfied is to allow yourself to eat until you feel satisfied! Satisfaction is a holistic concept in that it's essential to satisfy both mental and physical hunger to live a life of freedom. Satisfying yourself mentally means eating foods that bring you joy and participating in activities that improve your mental health.

Just like when the term "binge-eating disorder" is used in the context of eating disorder recovery, the term "emotional eating" is equally problematic. It suggests that food is not allowed to hold any emotional value and that taking pleasure in eating is immoral or wrong. But if food or eating wasn't supposed to be emotionally significant, why do delicious foods even exist? Why do restaurants exist? Why do holidays and recipe books exist?

When you consume something that you enjoy the taste of, your brain releases the neurotransmitter dopamine. Also known as the "motivational molecule" and the "habit-former," dopamine plays a vital role in the brain's reward system. This system is designed to reward the brain when you engage in activities that facilitate survival, including primal behaviors such as eating and sex. Interestingly, lower levels of dopamine have been found in neurodivergent individuals as well as those with eating disorders. Not only would further research on the role of dopamine in neurodiversity and eating disorders help understand why many individuals from these groups tend to show increased levels of guilt around eating, but it could help lay the foundation for more neurodiversity-affirming care. After all, change starts with awareness. You will learn more about rewiring guilt later in this book (and Module 8 of the accompanying course), so for now, I'll leave you with this: Taking pleasure in eating is not sinful. Our brains are designed to take pleasure in eating because eating is necessary for survival. And surviving is not a sin. So please, let's stop demonizing the term "emotional eating."

PART 4

RESTRICTION

13

RESTRICTION AWARENESS

What comes to mind when you hear the word "restriction"? You may associate it with cutting calories, categorizing certain food groups, or limiting amounts of food. But did you know that in some cases, eating *more* can also be a form of restriction? Or that forcing yourself to be productive is potentially another form? Just as there are different forms of hunger, there are different forms of restriction. In the previous section, you learned how thinking about exercise in certain ways is a disguised form of mental hunger. In like manner, your eating disorder will try to disguise restriction.

For so long, your eating disorder has been behind the wheel, like a parasite using your body and mind as its host. It's been sucking your energy for its own good, constantly influencing your every move. The first step to fighting off this parasite is becoming aware it even exists – you can't find a solution if you're not aware there's a problem! Recognizing the myriad of ways in which you restrict is the first step to building your awareness. The second step is redirecting the restrictive behavior by replacing it with a behavior you actually *want* to engage in. As with building any new habit, engaging in behaviors that support an abundance mindset rather than a restrictive one will feel scary. Yet, the only way for the new behavior to become easier – and eventually second nature – is to take action. Through consistent and intentional actions, you will neurally rewire your brain to know and trust the outcome of the life you were born to live.

14

TYPES OF RESTRICTION

Dietary restriction: the most obvious form of restriction, as you are directly restricting caloric intake. Letting go of calorie counting can be very difficult for those in recovery from an eating disorder, especially for autistic individuals. The ability to attach numbers to food provides a (false) sense of control, because the more you try to control calories, the more calories control you. If it's too overwhelming to completely stop counting calories, use counting to your advantage in recovery: instead of attaching a maximum amount to your daily intake, set a minimum and increase this amount in time increments that align with your level of desired challenge. Taking recovery-oriented action to exceed a particular number of calories will teach your brain that resources are not limited, which will eventually eliminate the need to count calories at all.

Portion control restriction: controlling and limiting your portion sizes to ensure you will not eat more than the amount you've allotted yourself. Some examples from my personal history of disordered eating include buying pre-portioned items (such as yogurt, ready meals, snacks, etc.), dividing items before eating them (such as slicing a banana in half first or only plating half a sandwich), using small bowls or plates and cutlery, and weighing and measuring food. To rewire your brain regarding portion control restriction, you must stop manipulating your portions. This means buying in bulk, eating out of different bowls and with different utensils, and cooking or ordering takeout instead of buying low-calorie frozen meals.

For autistic individuals in recovery from disordered eating, the aforementioned examples are a bit more nuanced. During my own journey to full recovery, I had a hard time veering away from the predictability of using certain tableware and utensils. Forcing myself to switch things up made my anxiety worse, which ultimately made it harder to eat. So, if you are autistic and in recovery, you may want to start by swapping your usual set of small items for a larger set and make that a part of your new routine. Even this switch will likely bring up fear, but remember what you learned earlier about fear: facing the fear provides your brain with knowledge of the outcome, and in time, you'll learn there isn't truly anything to be afraid of. The same approach goes for neural rewiring of any kind. Becoming aware of how you want to live and then taking actions that align with that desire provides your brain with plenty of data points to form habits that support a life of freedom!

Timing restriction: can be divided into infinite subcategories, but I find the most common forms of timing restriction manifest as allowing yourself to eat only a specific amount of (certain) food per day or per week or as saving (particular) foods for later. With timing restriction, it can be really easy to fall into the trap of thinking "it's not really restriction" because you may technically be allowing yourself all foods. However, if you are limiting the amount of food within a certain period of time (for example, not allowing yourself to eat bread more than once a day or only allowing yourself "cheat foods" on the weekends), you're restricting, which will keep you trapped in the grasp of mental hunger. To cease restrictions related to certain amounts of food within a certain time period, actively plan out how you will face your fears head-on. If you have rules around eating bread only once a day, make toast for breakfast and a sandwich for lunch. If you have a rule around eating pizza only on the weekend, order pizza in the middle of the week.

When it comes to saving calories for later in the day, you must take the same approach. If you find yourself eating small portions earlier and choosing to eat "healthy" throughout the day so you can "indulge" in the evening, assign minimum amounts for each meal at each time of day. And if you're worried that eating more throughout the day *and* feasting at night will cause you to go over your allotted amount of food, remember that's the whole point! There's no such thing as too much food. The more you eat, the faster you'll get out of energy deficit and the faster you'll overcome extreme hunger.

Avoidance restriction: avoiding food. Although you may be wondering how this is different from dietary restriction, avoidance restriction has its own section because it can present itself in subtler ways. One example of avoidance restriction is not allowing yourself to have a certain food in the house due to the fear that you won't be able to "control" yourself around it. Thanks to diet culture, this fear is common even in people who do not have eating disorders.

Instead of "protecting" yourself from overeating, however, the fear of not being able to control yourself around food is what precipitates bingeing in the first place. By conditioning your brain that you need to avoid or restrict certain foods, your brain perceives scarcity and is more likely to cause you to binge on them when they *are* around. So how do you break this cycle and learn to feel at peace around all foods? Allow all foods. When you stop giving your brain a reason to believe resources are scarce, it will stop believing they are.

Event restriction: a form of avoidance restriction that's all about creating an energy deficit in anticipation of an event where you won't have control over the food or exercise possibilities. Before any holidays, parties, or family gatherings, I would often increase my restriction and exercise to create a "buffer" for myself. Not surprisingly, I would decrease my intake and find subtle ways to incorporate extra movement at the event anyways, but it was the following thought that gave me relief: *just in case.*

Although knowledge that you have created a buffer may provide temporary solace (as with all restriction) during the event, the torture of having to plan out and worry about something that is supposed to be an enjoyable experience is totally not worth it. Plus, because any type of restriction is bound to be met by its equal and opposite reaction, the very foods you avoid before and at an event are likely going to be the very foods you end up bingeing on afterwards.

To beat your eating disorder to the punch (because food is so much more enjoyable when you are actually enjoying it rather than gorging in secret!) when it comes to event restriction, eat and move as you regularly would both before and after the event. If you find yourself tempted to behave differently due to anticipation anxiety, remind yourself that you can only create healthy neural networks around events if you act in a way that is aligned with the person you want to become.

Meal plan restriction: strictly adhering to a meal plan to ensure that you don't go over the amount on the plan. This was definitely one of the toughest forms of restriction for me to break! Meal plans can be a very helpful part of the recovery process, but they can also act as a barrier to becoming fully recovered. Let's be real: no normal eater walks into the kitchen craving a certain number of starches, proteins, and fats…

When I was still on a meal plan and wanted more food than was on the plan, I would excuse my restriction with the phrase "doctor's orders." As with all forms of restriction, your eating disorder will come up with any excuse to eat less. It's critical you disengage with the ED thoughts if you want to live a life of freedom.

Treat the meal plan as the bare minimum. If your healthcare providers tell you that eating more than your meal plan means you are becoming a "binge eater" or an "emotional eater," find a new provider. They're supposed to help you, not make recovery harder than it already is.

Comparison restriction: eating only when other people are eating and/or making sure to eat less than them. This can involve eating slower than others, encouraging others to eat just so you can eat as well, and exercising or moving if others are doing so. Just like meal plan restriction, comparison restriction was another habit I found super difficult to break. To free yourself from comparison restriction, you must rewire your brain in the same way you win the battle against all forms of restriction: do what you know you need to do to get out of energy deficit. Even if all humans ate and moved the same, our bodies would still all look different! If that doesn't illustrate how every person's energetic needs are unique, I don't know what does.

Compensatory restriction: using compensatory behaviors such as exercise, purging, or laxative use to make up for or earn food. Similar to how exercise hunger is a disguised form of mental hunger, compensatory restriction can be seen as a disguised form of dietary restriction. Even though you may not be eating less (you may even be eating more), the purpose behind the compensation is to negate the total number of calories consumed. This counteraction enforces perceived scarcity in your brain, resulting in increased mental hunger. To eliminate compensatory restriction, stop all compensatory behaviors! Yes, you may gain weight, you may get anxious, and you may feel an overall sense of loss as you challenge your eating disorder's rituals. However, this temporary discomfort is an investment in a life that's truly worth living.

Post-feast restriction: a form of compensatory restriction that involves eating less after an extreme hunger episode. Chances are, you're unfamiliar with the term "extreme hunger episode" – and that's because I totally made it up! I also like the word "feast." As I've alluded to previously, I don't favor terms such as "bingeing" or "overeating" because they hold a negative connotation, whereas feasting (i.e., honoring your extreme hunger) is a celebration of your body's healing. Whatever term you prefer to describe eating large amounts of food, it's essential that you do not restrict afterwards. The root cause of "bingeing" is restriction, so by restricting after a feast, you are simply setting yourself up to binge again. If your body senses abundance, it will not feel the need to feast. And how do you prove abundance to your body? Eat a lot of food. And after that, eat more food!

Volume eating: filling up on high-volume foods instead of (or before) eating the calorie-dense foods you are truly craving. Volume eating is another disguised form of restriction, because you are fooling yourself that you're eating more…but it's this very "fooling" that is the foolproof sign of restriction! By loading up on water and foods that aren't as calorically dense, you are attempting to reduce your hunger with the ultimate goal of reducing your caloric intake. Volume eating may help with physical satiation to a certain degree, but satisfaction isn't just physical; ensuring mental satisfaction is equally necessary when it comes to bEATing extreme hunger. Furthermore, vegetables and other high-volume foods are the last thing your body needs to come out of energy deficit. There's a reason you don't crave steamed broccoli during your extreme hunger episodes…so next time you feel the urge to eat a giant bowl of vegetables before allowing yourself that cookie, skip the salad and go straight for the entire pack of cookies. They'll be so much more enjoyable when your stomach isn't already full and bloated!

Safe food restriction: choosing the "safer" or "healthier" option of a food. This type of restriction can be more deeply ingrained in some people, not only because of diet culture but also if you are autistic. In today's society, which finds a way to label or shame every food out there, it's no wonder you may feel guilty for buying the supermarket-brand white bread instead of the organic, non-GMO, gluten-free, sprouted bread. During the course of my own eating disorder, I couldn't go without my daily dessert-flavored protein bar. When I tried one of the bars again after having eaten real cookies and pastries during recovery, I spit it out in disgust. You can try and trick your mind as much as you want, but your body knows that the light, dairy-free ice cream doesn't taste "exactly the same" as real, creamy, dairy ice cream. You can say "I can't even tell the difference!" as much as you want when you swap zucchini noodles in your favorite pasta dish, but your body sure as hell can. No matter what, everyone's gotta eat. Don't you think it's about time you started enjoying it?

The term "safe food" is quite common in the neurodivergent community as well, and its meaning may differ based on whether there is also an eating disorder present. I define a "safe food" in the context of being autistic as any food that makes me feel comfortable and, well, safe! Autistic individuals value predictability and routine, and knowing what they can expect from specific foods helps give them that. For this reason, many autistic individuals will always go to the same stores and buy the same brands so they can rely on what they already know and trust. If the individual is doing so to support their health and well-being, this isn't restriction; it's eating in a way that supports their health and well-being. In contrast, if an individual is buying a certain food repetitively out of fear that they'll overeat, gain weight, or "mess up" their diet if they do otherwise, the intention behind the purchase is rooted in fear and restriction – which is what you don't want if your goal is to bEAT extreme hunger. For this reason, it's essential you learn to distinguish between your ED behaviors and your autistic traits if you're an autistic individual in recovery. I would love to help you do this through 1-1 coaching (livlabelfree.com/coaching)!

Productivity restriction: constantly trying to be productive and limiting/avoiding any open or free time. Who would have thought productivity could be related to extreme hunger? Until I realized that constantly chasing "productivity" was a way in which I attempted to distract myself from mental hunger, I would have never guessed. Similar to how safe food restriction is influenced by diet culture, "being productive" is idealized by hustle culture. We're conditioned to believe that resting is "lazy" and a "waste of time." But what is the goal of being productive? *To achieve a certain outcome in a certain amount of time.* Right now, your goal is to come out of energy deficit, overcome extreme hunger, and free yourself from food obsession. So, the most productive thing you can do is rest, honor your hunger, and permit yourself the freedom to just *be*. A practical skill that was very helpful for me (and which I still use to this day) is blocking out "free time" on my calendar. Just like you nourish relationships with others by making appointments with them, you can nourish yourself by making appointments with yourself.

Monetary restriction: limiting the amount of money you spend. You may be wondering what money has to do with extreme hunger. As you learned, energy deficit causes the brain to believe resources (i.e., foods) are scarce. This perceived scarcity triggers your body to economize and act with caution when it comes to expending energy.

Acting as if money is a scarce resource further amplifies the notion that overall resources are scarce, which precipitates restrictive thought patterns. Just as you can only have an abundant mindset around food by eating an abundance of food, you can only have an abundant mindset around money if you prove to your brain that money is abundant.

P.S. I am not advising you to go out and spend money on anything and everything you can think of – that would only feed black-and-white thinking, the opposite of what you are trying to achieve! What I *am* saying is to give yourself permission to live a life in which your needs are being met and you are satisfying yourself in every sense of the word. You deserve to eat food that's not on sale. You deserve to buy new clothes that fit you. You deserve to go out and buy lunch with a friend. Doing so may feel "wrong" and scary, but that's only because your brain isn't used to it. The more you practice, the better your brain will understand that spending money is perfectly acceptable, which leads to an increased quality of life!

P.P.S. At the time of this writing, shifting my money mindset is something I am still practicing every day. I grew up with an undiagnosed autistic father who was unable to work, and my now single mother was the sole breadwinner of the family for as long as I can remember. In that context, money was often discussed as something to "spend wisely." I believe ultra-sensitive individuals are much more prone to internalize external worries, especially at a young age. Personally, I suspect this internalization led to my self-imposed responsibility for tasks that should have never belonged to a child, and my development of disordered eating behaviors was part of an overarching adaptive mechanism to grasp certainty in what I perceived to be unsafe circumstances. Today, I constantly remind myself that money is a tangible tool that can be traded for intangible value. For example, while spending money on a good book appears to be a material transaction, your return on investment is much more abstract. Reading the book fulfills you in metaphysical ways and leaves you with valuable insights that no price tag can encompass. Similarly, money put into experiences that enrich you on a deeper level is a cost that, in the long run, ends up giving you back more than the initial deposit. Although this mindset takes time to embrace when you've been conditioned to believe the opposite, money is not a scarce resource. The only resource that is diminishing by the minute is time. Being cognizant of this allows me to trade money for experiences that improve my overall experience of time, and it will allow you to invest in adventures that bring you closer to unraveling the life you were born to live.

15

REWIRING RESTRICTION

Your eating disorder is like a virus that uses your body and mind as its host, and it uses all your unique strengths – creativity, persistence, wit – to its advantage. Like any virus, an eating disorder cannot stand on its own. It must use a living organism to manifest, relying on your genetic material to multiply and spread. To become immune to your eating disorder's infiltrative ways, you must actively rewire your brain around all restriction. I know firsthand how tempting it is to skimp on butter or convince yourself to eat vegetables before believing that you "deserve" the sweet treat, but if you give your eating disorder an inch, it will take a mile. Once you stop giving it room, it will stop taking it!

However few or many of the mentioned forms of restriction apply to you, all restriction has one thing in common: it activates a scarcity mindset. In turn, this prevents you from living life to your highest potential – a life in which you are making your own decisions and marching to the beat of your own drum. So what does that life look like, and what steps are necessary to achieve it? That's where unrestricted eating comes in.

PART 5

UNRESTRICTED EATING

In the previous section, you learned all about restriction and why it's essential to rewire your brain's approach to restriction to bEAT extreme hunger. You now have a heightened awareness of the ways in which your eating disorder will try to drag you down with it, which is an essential mindset to have before taking action against the ED. Your brain doesn't learn by thinking the same thoughts; it learns by gaining knowledge and trust through the actions you take. To break the restrictive and limiting pathways in your brain and create novel and abundant ones in their place, you take steps that support an abundance mindset. One of these steps is taking an unrestricted eating approach to food.

16

WHAT IS UNRESTRICTED EATING?

First things first: What is unrestricted eating? Exactly what it sounds like: eating without restrictions. Now you may be thinking, "But Livia! That's impossible! I don't know any other way to think or live. I don't even know where to start!" Let me tell you a secret: you've already started. Just by picking up this book, you've already taken action. If you choose to enroll in my course and engage with the modules, you're already doing the work. I'm sure you've heard it before, but recovery doesn't happen overnight. Being fully recovered comes down to rewiring your brain, and rewiring your brain is the result of consistent action over time. So, by definition, an eating disorder isn't something you can switch on or off. What you *can* switch on or off is your mindset and your willingness to choose love and abundance over fear and limitation. No, you cannot make the fear go away or put the anxiety in a box and tuck it at the back of the closet, but you can choose to face the fear, knowing that doing so will result in providing your brain with new evidence. And the more new evidence your brain receives, the quicker it will create neural networks that support the life of your dreams.

If that life looks like having food freedom, ask yourself: *How would the free me be living?* Once you have your answer, go out and start behaving like that person. If you find yourself in a situation in which you are in doubt, ask yourself: *What would the free me do right now?* Once you have your answer, go out and own that situation. When you feel stuck and don't know if it's truly you or your eating disorder that wants to make a decision, ask yourself: *Which decision would the free me make?* Once you have your answer, go out and make that decision.

It is common to think you have to wait for some external event to happen before you can change or take action, but waiting for something outside of yourself is choosing to be a victim. If you want to own your life, you must take responsibility for it. Taking responsibility for your extreme hunger means honoring it without rules, judgment, or limitation. It means eating whatever you want, whenever you want. It means you must stop basing your food choices on others and actively disengage with diet culture when it presents itself. It also means eliminating the word "triggered" from your vocabulary. Why? Because being triggered is a choice. If you were planning to get pizza with a friend and they ordered a salad instead, you may feel tempted to skip the pizza as well, blaming this choice on your friend "triggering" you. However, the reason is insignificant; it will always be *you* who ordered the salad. Your friend didn't force the word "salad" to come out of your mouth, nor did they hold you down and threaten to hurt you if you ordered pizza. If you didn't order the pizza you really wanted, it means you allowed an external circumstance to make the decision for you – and as long as you allow yourself to be at the mercy of your external circumstances, you are choosing to be a victim.

But why should you stop being a victim of diet culture if everyone else is following diet culture? Why should you order pizza if ordering a salad is just as easy? Why should you want to stop thinking about food, weight, and body size since that's all anyone ever talks about? The more important question is: Why are you reading this book? If you're anything like I was, it's because you're sick of living a life that's controlled by external circumstances. Deep down, you want to be free from diet culture because diet culture fucking sucks. You want to be able to order pizza without guilt or shame because pizza is delicious. You want to stop thinking about food, weight, and body size because life is too precious to waste it thinking about things that don't excite you.

Taking an unrestricted approach to food is the golden ticket to living life to the fullest. When you start living in alignment with the person you want to become, you will most likely gain weight and you will most likely feel out of control. But that weight gain is symbolic of everything else you are gaining. And it's not *you* who's losing control – it's your eating disorder! Isn't that the very thing you no longer want controlling you? Your extreme hunger has only one goal: to get you out of energy deficit and pay back your energy debt. Unlike your eating disorder, your body has no hidden agenda – it's but a vessel for your soul to blossom. When you start eating unrestricted, you will be craving a lot of food…but this craving will dissipate over time. Your body has no reason to continue asking for heaps of food when you have paid back your energy debt, which means you also will not gain weight forever. But you're not at that point yet, so you may have some questions about unrestricted eating. Because I've been through the process and come out stronger and happier because of it, I'm honored to answer them.

17

JUNK FOOD

One of my biggest fears while going through extreme hunger was that I would become addicted to "junk food" if I followed my cravings. With the knowledge I have since gained about the influential nature of diet culture and fatphobia in our society, I'm not surprised by the commonality of this fear. It seems you can't look anywhere anymore without meeting yet another article titled "Study Shows Sugar Addiction Is Real" or "Why Junk Food Is Bad for You." What's truly "real" and "bad for you," however, are such articles!

When you hold particular beliefs – that certain foods hold moral value or that your worth is rooted in your ability to withstand certain types of food – you will seek out information to confirm these beliefs. At the same time, you will ignore or reject information that contradicts these beliefs. Known as confirmation bias,[1] this phenomenon doesn't apply just to food and eating; it manifests in all areas of your life. An everyday example can be found in politics. During presidential elections, people tend to seek information that paints the candidate they support in a positive light while dismissing any information that paints them in a negative light.

Confirmation bias is dangerous because it prohibits you from experiencing new opportunities and keeps you stuck in a limited mindset. If you believe you are "not sick enough" to seek help for your eating disorder, you will continue to come up with reasons why you should not seek help for your eating disorder. If you believe your mental hunger can't be trusted, you will continue to come up with reasons why you should distract yourself from it. If you believe that eating "junk food" will worsen your health rather than support your journey to overcoming extreme hunger and finding balance, you will continue to come up with reasons to avoid honoring your cravings. Bringing back a core lesson from chapter 2, these reasons for behaving a certain way act as the motivation to keep behaving that way.

In the words of the Buddha: all that we are is the result of what we have thought. The only reason you have an eating disorder is because you have conditioned your mind to think in a way that aligns with the beliefs of someone with an eating disorder. These beliefs are called limiting beliefs, as they limit you from living the life you so desire and deserve. Limiting beliefs are rooted in restriction and fear, which brings us back to the acronym from part 1 of this book: FEAR is False Evidence Appearing Real. Your limiting beliefs are what cause you to feel that you have "evidence" of a future worst-case scenario. But as you also learned, the only way to provide your brain with evidence of what will really happen when you act in opposition to your limiting beliefs is to face the fears head-on. If you want to be someone without an eating disorder, you must act in a way that aligns with the beliefs of someone without an eating disorder – juxtaposing this way with the way you've been acting for however long you've been abiding by your eating disorder's beliefs. So, to fend off your eating disorder's reasoning, you're going to need to know (and own) an even stronger reasoning.

Per usual, your clever body is one step ahead of the game. Before explaining how "junk food" plays into this game, let's switch over to the term "high-calorie food." Although your unconscious mind may still have negative associations with high-calorie foods, replacing the label around a certain type of food to something less biased and more factual reduces the negative load. You will learn everything you need to know about becoming label free in the last section of this book (and Module 8 of the accompanying course), but for now, let's focus on why no food or type of food can be labeled as "junk" or "unhealthy."

First, all food is energy. Whether you eat a salad or a slice of chocolate cake, your body recognizes incoming energy and will use that energy in ways it deems most efficient. When the body is in energy balance, it will ask for a variety of foods, including colorful produce and whole grains, but also sweet treats and more processed foods. When you are in energy deficit, the body can't be as loosey-goosey about incoming resources. Your top priority is survival, so your body will try to obtain the maximum amount of energy in the most efficient way possible. And what type of food contains the most energy? The foods you fear most! Nuts and nut butters, cereal, bread, cake, cookies, ice cream, burgers, pizza, pasta…all these foods contain a relatively high number of calories per unit of volume. Ever wonder why you never daydream about a bowl of lettuce or fear you'll "overindulge" on sliced cucumber? It's because these high-volume, lower-calorie foods are not what your body needs to come out of energy deficit.

Such a preference for high-calorie foods is an evolutionary mechanism to optimize your chances of survival. If you were truly in a famine (which is what your brain stem perceives), having access to, as well as the ability to consume, large amounts of nutrient-dense foods would literally save your life. So here's your biologically backed-up permission to honor all your cravings without restriction. Eating your fear foods will feel immoral and wrong, but that's exactly why they're your fear foods; you've conditioned your brain to believe consuming these foods is immoral and wrong. Eating large amounts of sugar, carbs, and fat will bring up thoughts that you are eating "unhealthy," but to overcome extreme hunger, eating large amounts of sugar, carbs, and fat is the most efficient way to *become* healthy.

Now, you may be thinking, "But what if I still crave all these foods once I am healthy?" Holding onto this fear is allowing your eating disorder to rule your life. By clinging to the belief that you will forever crave high-calorie foods, you will continue to come up with reasons why you should avoid these foods. But where has avoiding these foods gotten you? When you've paid back your energy debt and your body learns to trust you again, it simply has no reason to crave sugar and fat 24/7. I remember the first time I craved a salad after spending several months eating only sweet foods. I no longer desired sugary, fatty foods every moment of every day, as my body no longer *needed* these foods every moment of every day. As my body made its way into energy balance, I craved more colors of foods, and I also started craving more movement. Sweet treats and processed foods are still part of my daily eating habits, but they're no longer all I think about. I now have much more important topics on my mind!

18

NIGHT EATING

In my memoir *Rainbow Girl*, I share a scene that led to a panic attack. I describe how I used to spend the entirety of each day looking forward to my nighttime feast, which consisted of protein fluff topped with dried fruits, nuts and nut butter, chocolate, cookies, and everything else I wouldn't allow myself to eat during the day. Each night, I would present the food compilation to my family, waiting for their acknowledgment before I could finally satiate the day's buildup of mental hunger. On one occasion, I noticed my mom's eyes wandering during the acknowledgment moment. What followed was an explosion of anger as I blamed my mom for "ruining" my special event.

Looking back now, I see there was no rhyme or reason to my anger, let alone to the extent to which I placed my nightly eating routine on a pedestal. Yet at the time, it was what I lived for. My fantasies about allowing myself to eat without guilt and allowing myself to feel full could, in my mind, only be realized at night. During the day, I was so anxious that I often felt incapable of eating more than my perfectly portioned meals and snacks. Not to mention, I simply didn't feel physically hungry during the day due to my lack of interoceptive awareness. Since fullness is a very sensory experience that I used to perceive as uncomfortable and therefore "wrong," I avoided the sensation at all costs. Thinking about food 24/7 was how I paid the price.

In my years of coaching individuals to food freedom, I've learned I'm not the only one who found eating at night monumentally easier. Procrastinating mealtimes is a common way in which one obtains a sense of control. Completing tasks and checking items off your to-do list provides a hit of dopamine, which is further amplified when you finally allow yourself to eat. Along with reward circuits, habit-formation circuits are also relevant in the context of delaying eating. You may have heard the phrase "neurons that fire together wire together." Neuropsychologist Donald Hebb first used this phrase in 1949 to describe how pathways in the brain are formed and reinforced through repetition. When you repeatedly eat after a certain time or after you've completed a certain number of tasks, your brain becomes hardwired to associate eating with a time of day or level of task completion. On top of that, you have conditioned your brain to believe that food is more enjoyable when you save it for the evening. However, believing that you must wait until certain circumstances have been met before you can enjoy particular foods doesn't mean you have to hold this belief forever. As you learned in part 1 of this book, the brain's desire to cling to familiarity makes change one of the hardest tasks in human existence. On the bright side, using your brain's ability to change through commitment and intentional effort is one of the most powerful tools you possess. But why should you want to rewire your brain to eat earlier in the day anyways?

One of the most significant life lessons I've learned and keep coming back to is the idea that nothing outside of you can truly change you. Of course, external circumstances influence you and your actions all the time, but no amount of external conditions can change your mindset or your belief system. You do not choose to experience an eating disorder or endure a traumatic event, but you can choose how to respond to the happenings in your life. In the words of Viktor Frankl, a prisoner during Nazi Germany: "Everything can be taken from a man but one thing: the last of the human freedoms – to choose one's attitude in any given set of circumstances, to choose one's own way." You do not choose to be victimized, but you do get to choose whether or not you stay in a state of victimhood.

Personally, I became sick and tired of allowing external circumstances to rule my life. I became sick and tired of wasting my whole day thinking about food, just so I could enjoy a fraction of it in a realized food fantasy. I wanted to be able to crave something and eat it right then and there, rather than having images of that food swirl through my brain as I forced myself to focus on completing the tasks I deemed conditions of consumption. Restricting all day and waiting to eat until I had followed my movement ritual, tended to all of my digital notifications, and cleaned up my living space didn't truly give me control – these external circumstances controlled *me*. I wanted to identify with a person who was free in every sense of the word, and I could only do so once I started behaving like that person.

Choosing to live label free was the very change that permitted me to live life on my own terms. My attachment to external circumstances was a way in which I labeled my food behaviors: eating before a certain time was "wrong," and eating after I had completed a specific task was "right." I was a slave to everything beyond me, believing I would somehow be set free once I reached a tangible milestone. But the opposite was true. I was living in a self-imposed prison and could only be set free once I admitted to myself that I possessed the key all along.

At any given moment, you possess the choice to stop restricting, to stop delaying food, and to eat whatever and whenever you want. You will fear that these "new" actions will bring up anxiety and guilt, and in the beginning, they probably will – but the choice to engage in those thoughts is up to you. Your fears of taking actions perpendicular to your eating disorder's beliefs are only fears because the eating disorder's belief system has convinced you to live the way you are living now. But how you are living now is in a toxic entrapment. To cultivate the belief system of someone who possesses true freedom is to take actions aligned with your true self.

19

BREAKING THE CYCLE

Cultivating a life that's free of extreme hunger starts with breaking the restrict-binge cycle. One of the reasons I stayed stuck in the mental hunger games for so long was because I gave myself an ultimatum for ending my restriction: "Once I stop bingeing, I'll stop restricting." But it doesn't work that way. As you learned, it's not overeating that's the problem. The problem lies in not eating enough. Bringing back the metaphor of extreme (mental) hunger being Newton's Cradle, you understand that the more you swing towards restriction, the stronger your hunger becomes. By restricting the whole day to "make up for" last night's feast, you are simply setting yourself up for another feast – and, at the same time, strengthening the circuits in your brain to eat only in the evening.

Letting go of restriction and compensation after bingeing doesn't only support the formation of healthy neural networks, it also affects your sense of safety on a more primal level. Every time you honor your extreme hunger, you are providing your brain with the knowledge that resources are abundant. When you have provided your brain with enough of this knowledge, your brain finally has a reason to stop obsessing over food. At the same time, your nervous system (more on this in part 7) no longer perceives a threat and, thus, supports growth and healing. Unfortunately, the reality of going through extreme hunger doesn't often match this ideal scenario.

Every time I feasted at night, I would wake up the next morning and tell myself to "start fresh." I thought that if I just ate less the next day and managed to maintain my willpower and discipline for twenty-four hours, I would break the cycle and then eat "normally" again once "balance" had been restored. But can you guess what happened? Come evening, I would be so hungry that I'd shovel everything but the kitchen sink into my mouth. When I finally admitted that I held the key to break free from this restrict-binge prison, I unlocked the method that not only set me free from anxiety around food, but also set me free from extreme hunger. This key is eating an abundance of food. Not just after a binge, but *especially* after a binge.

By reinforcing abundance after I had proven it during a binge, I was strengthening my brain's belief that food would always be there. The more I provided my brain with the knowledge that resources were plentiful, the more reason it had to trust my body and its environment. So, in order to stop the restrict-binge cycle, you must stop restricting first. Once your body has no reason to binge, it won't! Of course, you have your own reasons (or rather, your eating disorder's belief system has its own reasons) for not eating in abundance – and a large part of that may have to do with the fear of weight gain and a changing body.

PART 6

WEIGHT GAIN

I used to believe weight gain was one of the hardest parts of the recovery process. That was until I was hit by the extreme hunger bomb. It was at that moment that I believed my body was broken. *I was already weight restored! My BMI was within normal range! If I gained more weight, I would probably gain weight forever!* It wasn't until I went through extreme hunger a second time – after losing weight for reasons completely unrelated to my eating disorder – that I realized it isn't the weight gain itself that's difficult; it's the associations you have with it.

As I've illustrated not only in this book but also in my memoir *Rainbow Girl*, mindset is everything. When we attach power to external circumstances, we become powerless against the external world. For years, I gave the grades on my school papers the power to decide whether I was a "good" student, I gave the food scale the power to determine how much I would eat, and I gave my eating disorder the power to control my life. Attaching your happiness to a number on the scale, a point on a BMI chart, or an arbitrary "target weight" prescribed to you by a health professional is giving these things the permission to steal your freedom – because freedom is to embrace your own way no matter the circumstances.

In this section, I will provide you with the knowledge and understanding of everything you need to know about weight, including the significance of BMI and target weights, what to do about your extreme hunger if you're already weight restored, the importance of overshooting your weight, and how long weight redistribution takes. You can follow along in Module 6 of the accompanying course (livlabelfree.com/course) for visual representations and action steps for coping with weight gain.

20

TARGET WEIGHTS

Do you have a goal weight or weight range you won't allow yourself to go over? Also known as a target weight or ideal weight, this number can be rooted in several factors, including the weight you were at before your eating disorder started, the weight associated with a certain BMI, or the weight prescribed to you by a healthcare provider. Your fear of weight gain has everything to do with the unpredictability of whether or not your weight will settle at or within a certain range. As with any external circumstance, giving a number, a point in time, a calculator, or a doctor the power to influence your eating behaviors is choosing to be a victim…and as long as you choose victimhood, you will not be truly free (more on this in part 8). Of course, releasing yourself from victimhood is easier said than done. In order to set yourself free, you will need a strong enough motivation to do so, and that starts with understanding why a goal weight can be one of the biggest barriers to bEATing extreme hunger and reaching full recovery.

Most of the time, healthcare providers base their calculations for your prescribed target weight on two factors: (1) your weight history and (2) body mass index. Before I explain the history of BMI and why this metric should be renamed the *bullshit measurement index*, let's talk about why you cannot be prescribed a target weight based on your weight history.

Your weight history can be broken down into several of its own factors, including the weight you were at before your eating disorder started and the overall trend of your weight growing up. The latter is often used in the case of early-onset eating disorders. For obvious reasons, using the pre-ED weight of someone who developed an eating disorder as a child would not be useful.

Although there is logic to the method of using one's weight history to determine what their potential future weight could be, several important factors are not considered. For starters, calculations based on your past weight don't take energy deficit or energy debt into account. As you learned in part 2 of this book (and Module 2 of the accompanying course), physical extreme hunger most often occurs as one is coming out of energy deficit, meaning after one has already gained some weight. Post-starvation hyperphagia will continue not until the body has come out of energy deficit but until energy debt has been paid back. Because your body is one of the most complex biological systems and is smarter than any conscious mind can comprehend, there is no way for any person (or thing, which is worth mentioning with the rise of artificial intelligence) to calculate what weight you will be at once your energy debt has fully been paid back.

As no number on the scale can reflect the status and repair of the internal damage done due to restriction, it is equally true that no number on the scale can reflect the mental implications during recovery from disordered eating. For example, if you are still obsessing over food and exercise – meaning you are still experiencing mental hunger – you are not yet at optimal health. Furthermore, having a number attached to your weight in recovery can cause your eating disorder to use that number as a means to disguise restriction, limiting you from reaching your fully recovered potential.

21

BMI

Along with your weight history, most health professionals use body mass index (BMI) to determine your "ideal" weight. BMI is a tool used all around the world to classify people into one of four categories: underweight, healthy, overweight, or obese. The calculation is based on the result of one's weight in kilograms divided by the square of one's height in meters. In mathematical terms:

$$BMI = \frac{\text{weight (kg)}}{\text{height}^2 (m^2)}$$

Using this simple formula, a person with a height of 1.60 meters and weight of 60 kilograms would have a BMI of $60/1.6^2 = 23.4$, placing them in the "healthy" weight range. But what if this person was engaging in eating disorder behaviors? What if they never permitted themselves to travel out of fear they would miss a workout? What if they were constantly thinking about food to the point where their life was passing them by? Along with physical factors including age, sex, body type, bone density, and muscle-to-fat ratio, *mental health* is not taken into account when determining someone's BMI. Essentially,

BMI is not scientifically reliable when it comes to determining one's state of health. So, if BMI is such an arbitrary measurement tool, why does basically every health professional still use it today? Let's take a little history lesson.

BMI was devised in the 1830s by Lambert Adolphe Jacques Quetelet, a Belgian astronomer, mathematician, statistician, and sociologist.[1] Notable is that Quetelet was nowhere near a medical doctor. During his work, Quetelet developed a passion for probability calculus that he applied to study human physical characteristics. He was best known for his sociological work aimed at identifying the characteristics of *l'homme moyen*, French for "the average man." This "average man" was Quetelet's representation of a social ideal, an ideal he believed was the mathematical mean of a population.

Quetelet's desire to quantify this social ideal prompted him to study human growth in the context of populations. These studies led to his conclusion that, other than the spurts of growth after birth and during puberty, "the weight increases as the square of the height." His equation was known as the Quetelet Index until it was renamed the body mass index in 1972 by Ancel Keys, an American physiologist who studied the impact of diet on health (and yes, this is *the* Ancel Keys that led the Minnesota Starvation Experiment, a study that illustrated the impact of malnutrition on overall well-being).

A very important aspect of the invention of BMI is the time frame in which it took place. Quetelet's studies were published during the early nineteenth century, when there were no computers, electronic devices, or calculators that could accurately assess or examine the human body like we can with the technology of today. He developed a system based on a simple math formula, while there is more than enough proof that no number can ever capture the complexity of our bodies and associated health issues. Furthermore, the 1800s were a boom time for racist science. Quetelet's studies were based solely on the size and measurements of French and Scottish men, meaning people of color, immigrants, and disabled people were not taken into account. Not to mention, zero women or members of the LGBTQIA+

community were part of this study. That is, the index was devised exclusively by and for white Western European men.

In addition to the exclusive group on which BMI is based, there are countless other indicators of health that BMI does not consider. Along with the aforementioned physical factors and BMI's negligence of mental health, there is one overlooked factor that overpowers any tangible ones: a trust factor. As mentioned throughout this book, the body gains trust in its environment by gaining knowledge of abundance. Your actions must reflect what you want your body to believe, meaning you must take actions that align with a life of abundance. For your body to believe that there is enough food and it doesn't have to worry about another perceived famine, you must prove to it that there is no famine. You do this by gaining weight and reaching a body fat percentage that gives the body permission to heal. In other words, to reach full recovery, it is essential to relinquish the bodily "ideal" that a man created over 200 years ago.

22

WEIGHT RESTORATION AND REDISTRIBUTION

In my years educating on the topic of extreme hunger, one of the questions I am asked most frequently is: "Why do I have extreme hunger even though I'm already weight restored?" And I get it – I had this exact same question when I was hit by extreme hunger. As I share in my memoir as well as earlier in this book, I didn't experience physical extreme hunger until I was at the highest weight I had ever been in my life. Already bursting with anxiety due to the physical discomfort that comes with rapid weight gain (not to mention as a highly sensitive autistic person), I believed my body was broken. Because I had barely experienced physical hunger cues until I was at a higher weight, I believed I had gained weight the "wrong" way, and I feared I would gain weight forever if I gave in to my hunger at that point.

I wish someone would have told me the onset of extreme hunger *after* gaining weight is a biological mechanism that must be embraced in order to fully heal. However, I was informed of the complete opposite: "You're weight restored, so you can stop gaining weight now." At the time, this statement was a celebration, and I was overjoyed. *I had made it! I had fully recovered! I could finally eat normally!* This was all great until my body started asking for an amount of food more than what I believed was maximally acceptable.

The question of why you have extreme hunger after being "weight restored" stems from fear: fear that you'll never stop eating, fear of endless weight gain, fear that you'll surpass your "ideal" weight range. Unfortunately, we live in a fatphobic, diet-culture-ridden society that demonizes weight gain beyond a certain point, that "ideal" weight prescribed by charts and formulas. But gaining weight beyond a certain point is often a critical aspect of reaching full recovery. To understand why, let's start by defining the term "weight restored."

Merriam-Webster Dictionary defines "restore" as *to bring back to or put back into a former or original state*. According to this definition, weight restored means that the former or original weight has been reached. However, when it comes to recovery from restriction, restoring weight (i.e., returning to the weight prior to your eating disorder) is often not enough. Aside from the fact that the disorder usually starts at a younger age and your weight as a child should be nowhere near your weight as an adult (in most cases), energy deficit and energy debt are overlooked when using an individual's BMI and weight history to define the weight at which one is "weight restored."

As you learned, weight provides no accurate measure of overall health, especially when you're looking at the impact of an eating disorder on your entire body. Your "weight" can be restored, but what about everything you cannot see? Your bones, your organs, your hormones, your thoughts…if you're still experiencing mental or physical extreme hunger, there are clearly parts of your body that are not restored! More accurate terminology is *health restored*, as this name embodies a holistic perspective. But even here, you must be careful, as the word "healthy" is often used without comprehensive context.

Even if you developed an eating disorder as an adult and were at a "healthy" weight before you started restricting your food, you will likely need to overshoot your previous weight in order to fully heal. Although I am not a huge fan of the term "overshoot," because it implies you are going "over" a weight that cannot accurately be predicted in the first place, I will use the term here for the sake of semantics. In a nutshell, body fat overshooting is the phenomenon of putting on more weight than your pre-ED or "target" weight in recovery. Of course, there are cases in which someone's eating disorder stemmed from dieting as a result of being at a much higher weight than was healthy for their specific body. For this reason, it's important to address set-point weights.

According to the set-point weight theory, each individual has a genetically programmed weight range that the body will try to maintain to ensure optimal biological functioning.[1] It explains why some people are naturally leaner, while others are healthier at a higher body fat percentage. In essence, the set-point theory vindicates body diversity and is the central pillar of the Health at Every Size movement, which proposes that ideal body weight has no one size. Thus, your ideal body weight is the weight range in which your body naturally settles when you are engaging in a lifestyle that supports optimal levels of health.

If you've made it this far, you understand that full reparation of energy debt is necessary to achieve your unique version of peak health. There's a lot of stigma around the need to eat a lot of food in recovery from restrictive eating, given that most people are unaware of how many countless calories you have to make up for. Not only do you have to make up for the energy you missed due to underfueling, but you need to consume additional calories to ensure that there is enough energy available to repair the internal damage caused by energy debt. These "extra" calories are all on top of the energy you already need to support your daily life, even if you had never restricted your food in the first place. So in a way, it's almost like you're eating for three people. Assuming your baseline caloric needs are 3,000 calories, eating upwards of 9,000 calories doesn't seem so absurd anymore, eh?

Just like you need to consume "extra" calories for an extended period to pay back energy debt, you will also need to carry "extra" body fat for a sustained duration to ensure optimal healing circumstances. You know how when babies are born, they're all cute and chubby and fat? Or how kids gain a lot of weight during puberty and then suddenly shoot upwards during their growth spurt? Biology has not done this for shits and giggles (although looking back at chubby baby photos may be funny now, ha!). Fat storage is absolutely essential for growth and repair of any kind. So no, you may not need to grow taller anymore, but all of the internal damage that you cannot see must have sufficient energetic reserves to be repaired.

Because being at a higher weight can feel extremely uncomfortable (it's new and unknown after all), you may wonder how long you need to stay at a higher weight. The simple answer is: as long as it takes for your body to fully pay off energy debt. Once it has repaired all internal damage and is no longer in energy deficit, the body has no reason to store additional energy. As posited by the set-point theory, your weight will settle within your body's ideal weight range. At the same time, your weight will redistribute to harmonize with your unique body type. When I fully committed to weight gain and allowed my body to do its thing, the weight mostly went to my face and abdomen area. I felt incredibly "disproportionate" and like my body had blown up in certain places. For this, too, there is a biological reason!

When you gain weight after a prolonged period of restriction, the body will initially store fat where it deems the fat most necessary: around your vital organs. Because fat is one of the most important energy sources when it comes to the repair of your heart, brain, and all the other biological systems affected by malnutrition, the body cleverly encases these areas to create a healing environment. Personally, I feared that my weight would never redistribute. But as with all fear, this belief was False Evidence Appearing Real. To discover the truth and embrace the free life I'm living today, I had to prove to my brain that my weight would settle and redistribute in my body's uniquely optimal way. I had to be patient and trust the process while my body did the rest. As soon as you give your mind and body permission to heal, they will. Unfortunately, it's the lack of clarity about how long it takes to reach your set-point weight that causes most people to go wrong.

What often happens is that someone will be doing really well recovery-wise: honoring all forms of extreme hunger, allowing themselves to rest, and accepting natural weight gain. When they continue to gain weight and then overshoot, however, unhelpful comments may start, and the recovering individual may feel uncomfortable and fearful about staying at this higher weight forever. The saddest part of all of this is that healthcare "professionals" may even recommend weight loss at that point because overshooting often results in a BMI that is higher than the "healthy" range. The result of this recommendation? The person who was doing so well in recovery will actively try to lose weight again. This is such a shame! After all they've done to challenge their eating disorder – both physically and mentally – and being so close to the finish line of full healing by weight overshooting, all of this hard work is undone the moment they start to lose weight again. Why? Because weight loss that has not been initiated by the body sets off alarm bells indicating that there are not enough resources available to heal. And what does the body do when it believes there is a lack of resources? It starts to conserve energy, and the whole process of distrust starts all over again. So, if you want to reach true, full recovery, you must lose the mindset of wanting to lose your overshoot weight. You must surrender to the process and have faith in your body's innate wisdom. Trust me, I know this is hard. But what's that cliché again? It isn't going to be easy, but it's going to be worth it!

PART 7

OTHER BODILY CHANGES

Along with weight gain, there are many other changes that will happen in your body. After all, a lot of repair work needs to be done! From healing digestive issues to managing hormonal shifts and more, this section of the book (along with Module 7 of the accompanying course) teaches you what to expect when you're expecting…expecting healing, of course :) Before diving into the mechanisms behind the changes you may encounter, it's important to have a basic understanding of your body's two main systems: the nervous system and the endocrine system.

23

THE NERVOUS SYSTEM

The nervous system is the electrical information highway of the body, carrying messages to and from the brain and spinal cord to the rest of the body. It consists of the brain, the brain stem, the cranial nerves, the spinal cord, the spinal nerves, and the enteric nerves.

Nerves are bundles of fibers made up of neurons. Because a collective group of neurons creates a nerve, neurons are often referred to as nerve cells. The communication between your mind and body is bidirectional thanks to different types of neurons, which can be classified as afferent or efferent depending on the direction in which the information travels across the nervous system.[1]

Afferent (= conducting inward) neurons, also called sensory neurons, are responsible for bringing sensory information from the outside world into the brain.

Efferent (= conducting outward) neurons, also called motor neurons, are responsible for carrying motor information away from the central nervous system to the muscles and glands of the body.

Both afferent and efferent nerve fibers work together to sense and respond to various stimuli, but they are not connected directly.

Instead, a third type of neuron – the interneuron or association neuron – acts as a relay between the two. Interneurons allow the brain to combine multiple sources of available information to create a coherent picture of the information being conveyed.

The nervous system can be subdivided into two major parts: the central nervous system and the peripheral nervous system.

Central Nervous System

The central nervous system (CNS) consists of the brain and spinal cord. It is the head controller of the body, interpreting incoming information, formulating appropriate reactions, and sending responses to the appropriate systems within the body. Everything we experience originates in the operations of the CNS.[2]

To give an example of your nerves in action, think about smelling a stinky sock. Everyone knows the horror of finding that lost sock in your hamper or your gym bag, or perhaps your friends placed it in your locker to play a trick on you. As soon as you smell the sock, you pull away…but what responses in the body cause you to take that action? When you smell the sock, your afferent neurons send signals about that smell up the spinal cord and into your brain, which then processes the information as disgust. Then, with the help of interneurons, efferent neurons send the information down your spinal cord and out towards the muscles, indicating what motion to perform – in this case, pulling away.

When you have a history of disordered eating, you have conditioned your brain to process certain information in a distorted way. When someone offers you a cupcake, for example, your brain creates an inventory of how you previously responded to similar information. If you have a history of saying "no" when someone offers you food, your brain uses this information to produce the response it deems most appropriate for the situation. In the case of being offered a cupcake, your efferent neurons will send denial-containing information to your voice and body language to indicate to the other person that you are denying their offer of the cupcake.

As you can conclude, the reason it's so important to equip your brain with new knowledge (i.e., saying "yes" to foods you have restricted for a long time) is to form new reference points for your brain. When your brain contains information that permits you to say "no" as well as "yes" to different types of incoming information, you regain the power over your own choices – you're no longer at the mercy of distorted habits.

Peripheral Nervous System

Whereas the central nervous system is made up of the brain and spinal cord, the peripheral nervous system (PNS) is made up of nerves that branch off from the spinal cord and extend to all parts of the body. The peripheral nervous system itself can be divided into two subsystems, one controlling external responses and one controlling internal responses.

Somatic Nervous System

Your somatic nervous system is the division of the PNS that governs the external activities of the body, including the skeletal muscles, skin, and sense organs. The somatic nervous system consists primarily of motor nerves responsible for sending brain signals for muscle contraction.[3]

Autonomic Nervous System

Your autonomic nervous system is the division of the PNS that governs the internal activities of the body, including heart rate, breathing, digestion, urination, and sexual arousal. It is made up of elements of the brain stem, some of the cranial nerves, and some of the spinal nerves.

Earlier in this book, you learned about interoception and its role in regulating inner cues. To put this understanding into context with the autonomic nervous system, interoception is dependent on a complex feedback system between sensors located in the viscera and the brain's interpretation of the visceral feedback (i.e., communication between neurons).

Historically, the autonomic nervous system has been further subdivided into two parts: the sympathetic nervous system and the parasympathetic nervous system. Many publications propose that these two systems oppose each other. Presumably, the sympathetic nervous system is associated with fight-or-flight behaviors, and the parasympathetic nervous system is associated with growth, healing, and restoration. This paired-antagonistic model was formalized in the 1920s.[4] Because most organs have innervations from both sympathetic and parasympathetic components, the paired-antagonism model evolved into "balance theories," which attempted to link an overall state of health with "autonomic balance."[5]

Although the antagonistic model of the autonomic nervous system is still prevalent in most textbooks and forms of health education, it fails to explain several aspects of human biology. A much richer and more all-encompassing explanation lies in the polyvagal theory.

Polyvagal Theory

Stephen Porges, a psychiatrist, neuroscientist, and author of the polyvagal theory, revolutionized our understanding of the autonomic nervous system by illustrating how it is much more complex than previously believed. In contrast to the "old model," which divides the autonomic nervous system into a sympathetic and a parasympathetic branch, the polyvagal theory breaks down the autonomic nervous system into not two but three unique branches: the sympathetic nervous system, the dorsal vagal complex, and the ventral vagal complex.[6]

The term "polyvagal" combines *poly*, meaning "many," and *vagal*, which refers to the nerve called the vagus. The vagus nerve is the longest and most complex of the cranial nerves, twelve pairs of nerves that can be observed from the ventral (bottom) surface of the brain. Also known as the tenth cranial nerve, nerve X, or CN X, the vagus nerve provides parasympathetic innervation to your neck, thorax (chest), and abdomen, directly influencing your breathing, heart rate, and digestion. In fact, over 80% of vagal fibers are afferent, meaning the vagus transports more sensory information from the viscera to the brain than the other way around![7] The vagus itself can be divided into a left and right branch, originating from two separate nuclei in the medulla in the brain stem: the dorsal motor nucleus of the vagus (DMNX) and the nucleus ambiguous (NA).

The dorsal vagal complex (DVC), or immobilization system, is the phylogenetically oldest of the three circuits and originates in the dorsal motor nucleus. Similar to how the brain stem is often referred to as the reptilian brain, the branch of the vagus controlled by the DMNX is also known as the reptilian vagus because it develops evolutionarily earlier than the rest of the vagus. Cells originating in the DMNX project to subdiaphragmatic structures (stomach, intestines, etc.), making the DMNX critical in the regulation of digestive polypeptides and gastric motility.[8] When there is no perceived danger, the vagal system services the needs of the internal viscera (e.g., heart, lungs, stomach, intestines) to enhance growth, restoration, and digestion. In threatening situations, however, these homeostatic processes are compromised. Overactivation of the DVC can cause dissociation, going numb, or blanking out – all characteristics of the "freeze" response. One of the earliest survival strategies of vertebrates is "death feigning," which can be observed as behavioral shutdown in humans. For this reason, the DVC is also known as the shutdown circuit. Inhibiting movement slows heart rate, decreases metabolism, and conserves oxygen, promoting adaptive responses such as diving in aquatic environments or death feigning in terrestrial ones. Unlike in reptiles, who can quickly shift back into homeostasis after long periods without oxygen, the cortex (outermost layer of the brain) in humans and other mammals developed at the cost of increased oxygen demands. To support this adaptation, the sympathetic nervous system evolved as mammals' first form of defense.

The sympathetic nervous system (SNS), or mobilization system, regulates your body's fight-or-flight response. It prepares the body for imminent danger by increasing heart rate to deliver more blood to areas of your body that need more oxygen. For example, if you needed to run away from a tiger, your SNS would ensure that more blood is pumped to your leg muscles. At the same time, your brain would receive more oxygen for increased alertness, and small airways in the lungs would widen to maximize respiration.

Last, the ventral vagal complex (VVC), or social engagement system, is the phylogenetically newest circuit. It originates in the NA. Whereas the cells originating in the DMNX project to subdiaphragmatic structures, cells originating in the NA project to supradiaphragmatic structures (i.e., larynx, pharynx, soft palate, esophagus, bronchi, and heart). In other words, the ventral branch of your vagus plays a major role in your ability to speak, eat, and breathe – all critical elements of social engagement. Additionally, the NA vagus has a strong influence on the heart. This "vagal brake" provides a neural mechanism to rapidly change visceral state by slowing or speeding heart rate.[9] Your vagal brake plays a critical role in regulating homeostatic processes. When the environment is perceived as safe, the vagal brake serves the internal viscera to facilitate growth, restoration, and digestion. It also inhibits the fight-or-flight mechanisms of the sympathetic nervous system, dampening the stress response of the hypothalamic-pituitary-adrenal (HPA) axis (further explained in chapter 27) and reducing inflammation by modulating immune reactions.[10] When there are environmental demands, the NA vagus can remove the vagal brake to activate the SNS. This removal supports fighting or fleeing behaviors in dangerous situations, but it also allows mammals to sustain exercise and attention, as well as to endure pain.

The three circuits are organized and respond to challenges in a hierarchy consistent with the Jacksonian principle of dissolution, which is the reverse of evolution. John Hughlings Jackson, an English neurologist, proposed that in the brain, higher (i.e., phylogenetically newer) neural circuits inhibit lower (i.e., phylogenetically older) neural circuits, and "when the higher are suddenly rendered functionless, the lower rise in activity."[11] Although Jackson proposed dissolution to exclusively explain changes in brain function due to damage and illness, the polyvagal theory proposes a similar model that is relevant for mammals in any state of health.

According to the polyvagal theory, the human nervous system has, via evolution, retained three neural circuits that are used sequentially in response to perception of the environment. In this hierarchy of adaptive responses, the newest circuit (VVC) is used first. If that circuit fails to provide safety, the older circuits are recruited sequentially. This means that the body will first respond to perceived danger through activation of the sympathetic nervous system. If the threat persists, the body will revert to its most primitive mode of self-defense: the DVC.

To understand the hierarchical use of the three circuits in context, let's use a war veteran as an example. Before a soldier goes to serve their country, they feel safe and are able to socially engage with their family, friends, colleagues, and anyone else they become acquainted with. When the soldier goes to war and is exposed to the dangers of war zones, their sympathetic nervous system activates to maximize their chances of survival; their heart beats faster, they become hyperalert, and they may even become severely wounded without realizing it until they've left the battlefield. One role of the SNS is to increase pain threshold (for instance, being unaware of a bleeding gash), as awareness of pain would compromise an individual's ability to efficiently escape danger. When longtime soldiers return from war, they often experience dissociation, depersonalization, and other symptoms commonly associated with post-traumatic stress disorder (PTSD).[12] The once outgoing individual becomes isolated and may be incapable of tasks they used to execute easily. The soldier's withdrawn behavior is a reflection of being in dorsal vagal shutdown – the body's last resort for self-preservation after excessive activation of the sympathetic nervous system.

Similar to how a soldier endures trauma when exposed to the dangers in a war zone, restriction causes trauma to the body. As you learned earlier in this book, your brain perceives a lack of adequate nutrition as a threat to your survival, which activates your sympathetic nervous system. This hyperarousal of your mobilization system causes many people with restrictive eating disorders to feel the need to move a lot, since your body believes you need to escape a danger zone.

Activation of the body's stress response also helps explain why anxiety is such a common comorbidity of eating disorders. One of my favorite quotes is "the opposite of anxiety isn't calm, it's trust." The reason you feel anxious is because you don't trust your environment – internally, externally, or both.

When you honor extreme hunger and finally give your body the nourishment and rest it needs, activation of the SNS is no longer necessary. The vagal brake is reinstituted with massive force, which can trigger the dorsal vagal complex. Feeling tired or foggy and wanting to be alone are all very common experiences in recovery from an eating disorder – your body is demanding time and space to heal itself. This is an incredibly costly process, especially after prolonged stress. Because the energy you consume needs to be directed toward the reparation of all the damage done by malnutrition, your ability to exert energy in ways not essential for healing is compromised.

According to the analytical rumination (AR) hypothesis, depression is an adaptation that evolved as a response to complex problems.[13] While this theory focuses primarily on the mental energy spared by turning inward, I believe the theory is holistically applicable. After all the energy you've spent on external demands, you've built up energy debt. The fastest way to repay that debt is by directing every morsel of consumed energy inwards!

So how exactly does the body repair itself when you're consuming high amounts of energy? The endocrine system plays a major role in restoring internal balance.

24

THE ENDOCRINE SYSTEM

Your endocrine system is your second bodily highway, working with the autonomic nervous system to elicit chemicals called hormones. When it comes to biology, the term "chemical messenger" is often thrown around, but it is important to understand that there are different kinds of chemical messengers.

Neurotransmitters are molecules produced by the nervous system that transmit messages from one neuron to the next via a process called neurotransmission. Neurotransmitters work locally and act very fast, as they only have to travel across the synaptic cleft – i.e., the space between two nerve cells, ranging from 20 to 40 nanometers. For reference, the average diameter of a human hair ranges from 80,000 to 100,000 nanometers.[1] So neurotransmitters are very, very tiny! Scientists have identified over 100 different neurotransmitters,[2] but these are some of the most commonly known neurotransmitters that will be discussed further in this book:

Serotonin

Dopamine

Gamma-aminobutyric acid (GABA)

Epinephrine (also known as adrenaline)

Norepinephrine (also known as noradrenaline)

Hormones, on the other hand, are secreted by glands in the endocrine system and travel through the bloodstream or extracellular fluid. Because they act on more distant sites in the body, hormones are slower to take effect and tend to be longer lasting. Some of the most commonly known hormones that will be discussed further in this book:

Ghrelin

Leptin

Insulin

Cortisol

T3 and T4

Estrogen

Testosterone

Melatonin

Similar to how a nerve is made up of nerve cells called neurons in the nervous system, a gland is made up of cells that secrete hormones in the endocrine system. There are over forty-three known glands in the human body, but the glands mentioned further in this book include the:

Hypothalamus

Pituitary gland

Adrenal gland

Thyroid

Ovaries (female)

Testes (male)

Pineal gland

Now that you know the basics, it's time to dive into the digestive issues and hormonal changes that may occur as a result of honoring your extreme hunger and healing your body!

25

DIGESTIVE ISSUES

I'm going to cut right to the chase: digestive issues are a pain in the ass (pun totally intended)! Not only are they painful, but they can be inconvenient and oh so embarrassing. During my own eating disorder recovery, my family used to joke about how awful it was when I farted. Boy, am I glad those gassy times are over! Along with gas, I experienced bloating (to the point where I had to buy pregnancy pants), nausea, cramping, acid reflux, on-and-off constipation, and diarrhea. If any of that resonates with you, keep reading….in this chapter, you'll learn the science behind why digestive issues occur and what you can do to heal them.

As discussed in part 2 of this book (and Module 2 of the accompanying course), the body will slow down or shut down processes that are nonessential to life when it perceives scarcity. Each and every part of your body requires fuel to function, which means that a lack of adequate fuel equates to inadequate functioning. If you are not eating enough, your body doesn't really need to digest a lot of food, so why would it waste its precious energy on digestive processes? Your body will slow digestion to conserve energy, using the limited energy it has available for more essential processes such as respiration and pumping your heart.

When you are in energy deficit, your body turns to your internal organs for fuel. To ensure your survival, your body will leach energy from your organs and muscles – including your digestive muscles. While actively restricting, you may not experience the effects of weakened digestive muscles because your digestive system doesn't have much *to* digest. When you start eating more and providing your body with evidence that food is abundant, however, that's when you start to feel like you're being kicked in the pants.

Your body digests food through the process of intestinal peristalsis – a series of wavelike muscle contractions that move food through the digestive tract.[1] When these muscles are too weak to contract as they normally should, food may sit in your stomach for a longer period of time. This is called gastroparesis or delayed gastric emptying.[2] Of course, you only experience the symptoms accompanying gastroparesis – nausea, cramping, bloating, farting, etc. – when there's an abundance of food sitting in your stomach. Ahem, thanks extreme hunger!

Digestive issues can be a super discouraging part of the recovery process because you may feel like you're being punished for challenging your eating disorder's restrictions. But trust me, digestive issues are part of the healing process. By pushing through the uncomfortable symptoms and continuing to eat, you are literally pushing your body to become stronger again. By continuing to challenge the deeply ingrained rules in your brain, you are training your body to fight off the parasite of an eating disorder. And by eating larger amounts of food, you're literally training your digestive muscles! Just like you need to give your brain a reason to form new neural networks by taking actions that align with your healthy self, you need to give your digestive system a reason to become stronger again by eating.

The same goes for healing acid reflux. At one point in my recovery from an eating disorder, I was diagnosed with GERD: gastroesophageal reflux disease. Someone with GERD will experience unintentional vomiting, reflux, and/or heartburn after they have eaten.[3] At the time, I was grateful my problem had a label – I knew what was wrong! But looking back with the label-free perspective I have now, my doctor's almost instantaneous diagnosis of GERD without inquiring about my health history goes to show how fucked up the healthcare system is. As a result of that appointment, I was sent home with two prescriptions for antacids and the recommendation to "not eat at least three hours before bed."

With my current knowledge of the human body and how it responds to stress, I am shocked by the way that doctor (and many others) handled my situation. I didn't have too much stomach acid, I had too much stress and too little muscular strength. The real cause of unintentional vomiting during recovery from restriction has to do with the mind-gut connection (more on this in a moment) and the lower esophageal sphincter (LES). Normally, the LES opens as you eat and then closes to prevent stomach contents from traveling back up. However, what happens to muscles when you've been malnourished? That's right: they weaken and do not expand and contract as they should. This is the same with GERD: the LES weakens, meaning it won't expand and contract as it should. So, when you start fueling yourself adequately, you are much more likely to experience GERD-like symptoms.

***

Aside from weakened muscles, unintentional vomiting and other digestive issues are impacted by the state of your nervous system. The latter became crystal clear to me when I went into energy deficit and eventually experienced extreme hunger a second time, after I had fully recovered from my eating disorder.

As I share in my memoir *Rainbow Girl* and in a Liv Label Free Podcast episode released in November 2022, moving to the other side of the world by myself was challenging in every way possible. I had embarked on my journey from the Netherlands to California full of excitement and ambition, but that adventure turned out to be a far greater obstacle than I could have ever foreseen.

San Francisco is one of the most expensive cities in the United States (if not the world) and earning enough to cover my monthly costs – just the basics including rent, utilities, and groceries – proved to be a lot harder than I thought. I had only taken Liv Label Free full-time during the summer of 2021, and my income was not sufficient from clients or brand partnerships alone. To ensure I could pay my bills, I buried myself in work. I believed that as long as I was helping others, it would be worth it. Right? My body didn't seem to agree.

A few months after settling into my studio apartment, I started unintentionally throwing up. I had three part-time jobs at this point, leaving me with no time to recharge or build any kind of social life. The 6,000 miles and nine-hour time difference from my family in the Netherlands didn't help much either.

As the months progressed, the vomiting got exponentially worse and I started losing weight. I received negative comments on social media, including "you're becoming anorexic again," "you're relapsing," and "you are a trigger to the ED recovery community." Although I've developed much resiliency when it comes to owning my truth, these comments hurt. I had worked so hard to fully recover from my eating disorder, and receiving discrediting comments – from the very population I was trying to help, at that – felt like a stab in the heart. But I had to keep fighting, no matter what.

I continued overworking, drowning myself in distraction to hide from the loneliness and fear. I was striving for financial security and believed that all my health issues would resolve once I felt financially safe. But the safety I thought I would achieve with a certain amount of money was an illusion. As Eckhart Tolle writes in his book *A New Earth*, "the ego wants to want more than it wants to have." What this means is that the ego – or your identity of self – will continuously strive for a state of wanting, naturally resulting in an everlasting sense of dissatisfaction. After all, desire does not exist without lack. So, in an effort to fulfill the ego's desire for more, your mind tricks you into thinking that salvation can be found in external circumstances – or what I've come to refer to as labels.

Throughout my life, I've been labeled many things. Being labeled "hopeless" and "too complex" by healthcare professionals and inflicting the labels "vegetarian," "vegan," and "foodie" (among others) on myself, I've tried to fulfill a variety of external identities. But the more I identified with something external – the more I sought to find myself beyond myself – the more I lost myself. It was only once I became Liv Label Free and admitted that nothing outside of me could save me that I became truly free. This realization was scary, as it meant I could no longer be a victim to my circumstances. I had to take responsibility for my health, which, after all, is the only true form of wealth.

So, when I started experiencing other symptoms as a result of continued weight loss, including heart palpitations and insomnia, I decided enough was enough. I had to start prioritizing my well-being and take responsibility for my healing – nothing outside of me was going to do the work. I gave myself permission to move back home and spend time with loved ones, which resulted in an almost immediate end to the vomiting. Uncoincidentally, it was on that very day of granting myself permission that I experienced my first extreme hunger episode in years. I knew even then that these parallel events had something to do with the mind-gut connection, but with the increased knowledge of the autonomic nervous system and polyvagal theory I possess today, I have no doubt about it. I share this story so I can now teach you how to heal your digestive issues with that same understanding.

As I mentioned, my unintentional vomiting was the result of being in an almost constant state of stress. In polyvagal terms, I was switching between the SNS and DVC, feeling either hyperaroused or immobilized at any given moment. Naturally, these survival states inhibited the proper functioning of my VVC, which supports social engagement. The fact that I felt I didn't even have time for social interaction during my period of overworking and overwhelm? No coincidence!

Vomiting and other types of digestive dysfunction are part of the body's adaptive response to danger. When the body perceives a threat, it will first activate the sympathetic nervous system to fight or flee. Activation of the SNS stimulates your adrenal glands to secrete adrenaline and noradrenaline, which function as both neurotransmitters and hormones. Not only do these chemical messengers increase the flow of oxygen to areas of the body that can help you escape danger, but they also suppress feelings of pain.[4] Remember our example of the soldier at war? They didn't feel the bleeding gash in their stomach until they had safely landed in the hospital, reverting to their DVC after too much activation of the SNS. The adrenaline rush allowed them to quickly escape the danger zone without being distracted by the pain from their wound. The same is the case when it comes to recovery from an eating disorder. When you fully honor your body's hunger and need for rest, you will likely feel very tired and your body may begin to hurt. Although it may seem that recovery brought on this sudden suffering, it was there all along… but because your body felt it was in danger (rightly so: it was!), your pain response had been dampened.

As you can imagine, digestion is your body's last priority in a life-or-death situation. Whether you need to run away from a tiger or pretend you're dead, energy expended on digestion could be the actual death of you. Although you may think healing from restriction is completely unrelated to a tiger attack or being drafted to war, remember that your body perceives restriction as a threat. And when the body perceives a threat of any kind, your most primal biological mechanisms activate – whether you like it or not.

So, if digestive issues can be caused by both energy deficit and a hyperaroused or an immobilized state, how can they be healed? By getting out of energy deficit and bringing your nervous system back into the ventral vagal state. These two "solutions" to healing are two sides of the same coin, as you obviously cannot come out of energy deficit if your body is unable to properly digest food. At the same time, coming out of energy deficit – which you do by providing your body with evidence that food is abundant – informs your brain that you are not actually in a threatening situation and thus, neither the SNS nor the DVC needs to be activated. One of the easiest, most effective ways to activate your ventral vagal complex is to stimulate your vagus nerve by taking slow, controlled breaths. You may have heard of this breathing method before in regard to easing anxiety, and for good reason. Deep breathing increases the supply of oxygen to your brain, signaling safety (trust) and permission to (literally) rest and digest.

* * *

Another two-sided coin that can aid in not only healthy digestion but also better mental health is increasing food variety. Of course, you know your own needs best when it comes to how many different foods you feel comfortable eating. Autistic people tend to have more difficulty with eating a variety of foods, so remember to challenge yourself within your personal limits. Recovery isn't a race or a competition. It's about showing up consistently to put in the work – whatever that looks like for you. Increasing food variety doesn't have to mean eating a new exotic food at every meal or going out to a new restaurant every day. It can be as simple as having pasta as your carb source for dinner one night and having potatoes the next. Or making a banana protein smoothie for breakfast one morning and having a banana yogurt bowl the next. What's most important is that you don't cut out foods, as restriction of any kind will send your body right back into a stressed state.

Before my GERD diagnosis, I was diagnosed with irritable bowel syndrome (IBS) during the course of my eating disorder. Just like GERD and gastroparesis, IBS falls under the umbrella of functional gastrointestinal disorders (FGIDs), also known as disorders of the gut-brain interaction.[5] As the name suggests, FGIDs correlate to dysfunctional communication between the brain and gut – in scientific terms, dysfunction of the gut-brain axis.

Simply put, the gut-brain axis (GBA) is the two-way biochemical signaling that takes place between the gastrointestinal tract and the central nervous system.[6] The axis consists of multiple connections, including your gut microbiome, your immune system, and (not surprisingly) your vagus nerve. This means that dysregulation in any of these pathways can result in digestive problems.

You've already learned about the importance of the vagus nerve in digestion, so what about your gut microbiome and immune system? Just as restriction triggers your biological threat response to fight, flee, and eventually freeze, it also triggers imbalances in your gut microbiome. In turn, this leads to decreased immune function, increasing the chance of malabsorption and infection.

When you consume a limited diet, the diversity of bacteria in your gut decreases. Countless studies have demonstrated that the more diverse your diet, the more diverse your gut microbiome and thus the more resilient it is to perturbations.[7] To elaborate, species-rich intestinal communities are better able to fight off pathogens because specialized bacteria are equipped to exclusively target the invader. One study published in *Nature* illustrated how malnourished children who had significantly lower diversity of gut microbiota were more prone to developmental delays and long-term health consequences resulting from infection.[8]

Thankfully, transitioning to a diet rich in macronutrients and micronutrients from varied sources can restore a healthy gut microbiome, indirectly strengthening your immune function. Therefore, it's essential that you prioritize eating a wide variety of foods in recovery and don't give in to the temptation to cut out certain types of foods or entire food groups. And before you think "Oh no, this means I have to eat healthy!" remember what you learned in chapter 17 about "junk food": eating high-calorie foods is the most efficient way to come out of energy deficit. Restoring energy balance is your body's first priority. When the time comes, your body will naturally crave more whole foods and, in due time, restore microbial balance.

As I explain in my memoir *Rainbow Girl* (I know I keep referencing that book, but that's because it's my entire life story!), I was put on a low-FODMAP diet when I was diagnosed with IBS. The low-FODMAP diet is a protocol that limits the amount of FODMAPs an individual consumes. FODMAP stands for fermentable oligosaccharides, disaccharides, monosaccharides, and polyols. FODMAPs are short-chain carbohydrates (sugars) that have an osmotic effect (increasing the amount of water in the bowel) and are easily fermented by bacteria, meaning high consumption can lead to bloating and gas.[9]

At the time of my low-FODMAP prescription, I was desperate for relief. Not to mention, I now had an excuse to follow a strict diet...I mean, a *professional* recommended it! Eating a low-FODMAP diet did initially relieve my symptoms, but not for long. Understanding of the gut microbiome helps explain why.

Just as you need to train your digestive muscles to move food through your system, you need to train your gut to flourish. A variety of bacteria (and thus, the ability to tolerate a wide variety of foods) will only populate your gut if you give it a reason to. By eating a limited diet, your body has neither resources nor reasons to optimize its internal environment – that would be a total waste of energy! However, when you provide your body with an abundance of calories from different sources, you're creating an army of specialized soldiers within your body. The more uniquely trained soldiers you have, the stronger the entire army becomes against potential threats.

I know firsthand how tempting it is to seek the temporary relief that comes with cutting out certain food groups, but it's just not worth the long-term consequences. Research on the low-FODMAP diet shows that restriction of non-digestible carbohydrates generally has opposite effects, decreasing the abundance of "good" bacteria and increasing the abundance of "bad" bacteria in the gut. While I always hesitate to use labels such as "good" and "bad," I choose to use them with elaboration here, as that is how bacteria are commonly distinguished.

Generally speaking, good bacteria are types of bacteria that are known to have positive impacts on overall health. You have most likely heard of probiotics before, which are live strains of "good" bacteria present in fermented foods like yogurt, kefir, kimchi, and tempeh. Two popular examples of good bacteria are *Bifidobacterium* and *Lactobacillus*. Both are probiotics present in your intestines that help digest fiber and strengthen your immune response.[10] An example of a "bad" bacteria is *Bilophila wadsworthia*. And before you think this bacteria must be avoided at all costs, the presence of *Bilophila wadsworthia* is actually part of a normal human gut![11] In fact, a healthy gut comprises billions of different good and bad bacteria. Because we need both, neither are truly good or truly bad – as with everything in life, it's all about maintaining an optimal ratio.

In a systematic review observing the effects of the low-FODMAP diet on human gastrointestinal microbiota composition, researchers observed a decrease in the abundance of *Bifidobacterium* and *Lactobacillaceae* and an increase in *Bilophila wadsworthia* in the intestines of subjects who followed a low-FODMAP diet long-term. Furthermore, the initial reason for going on the low-FODMAP diet – to relieve digestive distress – actually led to worsening of the issues, including the development of several intestinal diseases.[12]

Although you may find some relief by eliminating certain foods or food groups from your diet, growing evidence shows that this relief may not even be due to the actual removal of the food. You've most likely heard of the placebo effect before: a beneficial effect produced by a placebo or "dummy" treatment, indicating that the changes are a result of the patient's belief in the treatment rather than the treatment itself. There's also the *nocebo* effect, which is the opposite of the placebo effect. As you can likely conclude, the nocebo effect takes place when a patient develops negative side effects or symptoms from believing that the nocebo is causing harm. In the case of gut issues and elimination diets, certain foods are the nocebo and the elimination diets are the placebo.

Upon being diagnosed with IBS and learning that specific foods (such as gluten, dairy, and processed sugars) exacerbated my symptoms, I rationalized the long-standing beliefs instilled in me by my eating disorder and by diet culture. In order to feel "normal," all I had to do was cut these foods out of my diet! But then why had I been eating all these foods for years with no issues? Why is it that I can now eat all those foods with no issues? Because it wasn't the actual food causing the issue. It was the *belief* I held around the food. And I'm not the only one who's experienced relief by eating the very foods that I once believed were causing me harm. According to the results of fifty published clinical trials, the placebo response rate in people following the low-FODMAP diet is as high as 84%, meaning 84% of IBS patients reported feeling better simply by *believing* they were receiving a treatment that would make them feel better. A similar result occurred in patients suffering from functional dyspepsia, another FGID common in recovery from disordered eating that is characterized by feeling overly full, bloated, and nauseous.[13]

The undeniable results of believing that certain actions will make you feel better and others will make you feel worse is one of the most powerful illustrations of the mind-gut connection. Remember what you learned about the gut-brain axis and the importance of a healthy vagus nerve and gut microbiome? Well, now it's time to dive into just how important that vagus and gut microbiome really are when optimizing both your mind and gut health!

Surely, you've heard the phrases "go with your gut instinct" and "have butterflies in your stomach" before. These expressions refer to the innate wisdom of your gut, which is regulated by your enteric nervous system. The enteric nervous system (ENS) is a complex network of nerves embedded in the walls of your gastrointestinal system. These nerve circuits are so extensive that the ENS is able to function independently from the central nervous system (CNS) while still communicating with the CNS through the gut-brain axis.[14] The ENS is often referred to as the "second brain" or "gut brain" due to the enormous number of neurons hosted within the system. In fact, more neurons are said to reside in the human gut than in the entire spinal cord![15]

The enteric nervous system uses the same chemicals as the brain, and growing evidence shows that gut microbiome impacts mood and behavior. For example, serotonin is a neurotransmitter correlated to a positive mood. Most people associate serotonin merely with a brain chemical, but nearly 95% of the body's serotonin is produced in the gut![16] Another example is dopamine, a neurotransmitter associated with motivation and reward, of which more than 50% is synthesized in the gut.[17]

If you are autistic, have ADHD, or have other connections to neurodiversity as an individual or a carer of someone with a unique brain, you are right to wonder about the impact of gut health on mental state. Whereas different forms of neurodiversity are usually addressed with therapies or strategies targeting what is perceived as an exclusively mental condition, a holistic approach that includes focusing on other bodily systems is often bypassed. To take the previous examples of serotonin and dopamine, autistic individuals are commonly found to be lacking in these two molecules. Suddenly, the gut issues experienced among the neurodivergent population make a lot more sense, eh? Furthermore, digestive distress may be more common among the neurodivergent because of the overall state of the nervous system. Navigating a world that wasn't built for you can result in a constantly alternating state of fight, flight, or freeze, of which diagnosable mood disorders such as anxiety and depression are a frequent result.

But even if you're not neurodivergent, a deeper understanding of the nervous system is just as important on your recovery journey. The main takeaway is this: you must focus on healing the body from an all-encompassing, inside-out approach to internalize health on every level. Of course, speaking about your struggles, your goals, and who you want to be is a critical aspect of becoming that person, but calming your nervous system and nourishing your gut are two equally important parts of the puzzle.

A growing body of research has found that increasing levels of "good" bacteria in the gut has a direct impact on neurotransmitters in the brain. In a 2020 study, researchers worked with rats subjected to maternal deprivation, making them naturally stress-sensitive. After treatment that involved administering a probiotic mixture, the rats' brains had increased dopamine and serotonin levels and a decrease in anxiety levels.[18] In another study observing the probiotic effects in a rodent model of autism, researchers measured increased levels of gamma-aminobutyric acid (GABA) – an inhibitory neurotransmitter that produces a calming effect – following treatment with several *Bifidobacterium* and *Lactobacillus* strains.[19]

What does all this research tell us? That healing lies on a level far deeper than our conscious awareness and that our "second brain" plays a key role in regulating our "head brain," therefore directly impacting our thoughts and behavior. Important to note is that the few studies mentioned here are just the tip of the gut-brain research iceberg!

Because the gut and brain are connected bidirectionally through pathways including the vagus nerve, taking a holistic approach is the most effective way to heal. This includes engaging in recovery-oriented actions such as challenging your fears, investing in tools such as coaching and courses, and rewiring your brain to create new associations with food, exercise, and your body. As discussed earlier, it's equally important to bring your nervous system into a calm state and eat an abundance of foods to help your gut flourish.

26

HORMONAL CHANGES

Aside from weight gain, so far you've learned about the bodily changes that happen in conjunction with the working of your nervous system. Now, it's time to discuss the hormonal shifts you can expect on your healing journey and how to navigate them.

When people think about changing hormones, they often immediately think about anything that has to do with reproduction. "They're just being hormonal" is a phrase I'm sure we've all heard someone say to describe an individual on their period. But hormones go way further than just reproductive health. They play a key role in your energy, mood, metabolism, sleep, and so much more! So what are hormones exactly? Hormones are chemical messengers secreted by your endocrine system and responsible for regulating different systems in the body. They are composed of various nutrients such as cholesterol, amino acids, and fats, and they travel through your bloodstream or extracellular fluid. In contrast to neurotransmitters, which act locally and quickly, hormones act on more distant sites in the body and tend to have longer-lasting effects. Most hormones come into contact with all of your cells, but each hormone affects only its specific target cells. This means that a certain body part can be affected by a specific hormone only if that body part has receptors for that hormone. If it does, those receptor cells are the target cells for the hormone. Estrogen, for example, is a hormone secreted by the ovaries and has target cells in the uterus, breasts, bone marrow, and brain.[1]

As with all bodily systems, the endocrine system requires fuel to function. Because the endocrine system plays such a vital role in several biological processes, including respiration, metabolism, reproduction, sensory perception, movement, and growth, energy deficit has serious ramifications for the working of your hormones. When you are malnourished, the body must become very selective in which hormones it secretes. Just as your body will not send out physical hunger cues if it does not trust you to respond to them, your endocrine system will not elicit adequate amounts of hormones if it does not deem them necessary for your survival.

When you start to come out of energy deficit and build trust with your body, your hormone levels will fluctuate. This can result in a myriad of confusing changes, including mood swings, aches and pains, and temperature changes, just to name a few. What role do hormones play in these changes, and how can you optimize healing? First, it's important to remember that your body is an integrated system that requires a holistic view to (even partially) understand. Even though us humans have been studying our anatomy for thousands of years and there have been incredible scientific breakthroughs, there's still so much we don't really know! Throughout the following sections, you'll learn scientific reasons for certain hormonal occurrences and gain tools to better navigate them. However, it's crucial to note that the endocrine system is too complex to trace hormonal imbalances to dysfunction of a single gland or its produced hormones. All your hormones work in concert to optimize your body's chances of survival, meaning an open and curious mind is necessary to absorb and internalize this symphony of science.

* * *

I had mixed feelings when I committed to full recovery from my eating disorder. A part of me was fearful – who would I be without the identity of the ED? – while a greater part of me was excited. I was going to embark on a journey that would lead to freedom; who wouldn't be excited about that? My elation regarding this endeavor proved a reality once I finally gave myself permission to do all the things I'd wanted to do for years. However, it didn't take long for the fear, worry, and regret to sink in. When I hit the highest weight I'd ever been and my extreme hunger showed no signs of stopping, I started researching leptin and insulin resistance. Had I damaged my body beyond repair? Could I no longer detect fullness because my fat cells were broken? Had I developed a sugar addiction with all the sweets I'd been eating? If you resonate with any of these fears, let's have a little chat about the hormones that play a role in hunger and fullness.

Ghrelin

Ghrelin is a hormone that is mainly produced in the stomach when it is empty. Ghrelin is often referred to as the "hunger hormone" because it regulates appetite and increases food intake. When the body believes it's time to eat, ghrelin cells in the stomach secrete the hormone, triggering a rise of ghrelin in the bloodstream. Ghrelin acts on the hypothalamus, where it binds to specific receptors known as growth hormone secretagogue receptors (GHSRs). When ghrelin binds to GHSRs on neurons in the hypothalamus, it triggers a series of biochemical reactions that ultimately result in food-seeking behavior.[2] One of these reactions is the release of neuropeptide Y, which stimulates appetite and prompts food intake.[3]

Leptin

Leptin, on the other hand, is a hormone responsible for signaling satiety. The main function of leptin is homeostasis regulation. To elaborate, leptin helps prevent hunger and regulate energy expenditure so your body doesn't initiate hunger when it doesn't need additional energy.[4] Unlike ghrelin, which is produced in your stomach, leptin is produced by fat tissue, making the amount of leptin in your blood directly proportional to the amount of body fat you have.⁵ If your body fat percentage is lower than your body's natural preference, you will have lower levels of leptin and thus you will require more food to feel satisfied. This is the key reason that weight gain is often an essential part of the recovery process, as it helps to restore healthy leptin levels. It's also why eating high-volume "replacement" foods doesn't truly curb appetite, because appetite isn't the problem. Your body craves high-calorie, nutrient-dense foods because these foods support necessary fat accumulation, which supports normal leptin levels. So as long as you're not feeding yourself with foods that will actually satisfy you, you won't be satisfied!

Similar to ghrelin, leptin travels through your blood and acts on the hypothalamus. When you have eaten enough to support your body's energy demands, leptin binds to hypothalamic receptors, activating or inhibiting neurons and neuropeptides that suppress appetite and increase energy expenditure. If ghrelin causes the release of neuropeptide Y, what impact does leptin have on this appetite-stimulating molecule? You guessed it: leptin inhibits neuropeptide Y, a mechanism that ensures your body stays within its set-point weight range.⁶

If you're reading this as someone in a larger body, you may be wondering if there's something wrong with your leptin levels; why do you have extreme hunger if you already have enough fat? Are you leptin resistant? It's important to understand exactly what leptin resistance is before drawing fear-based conclusions. As the name suggests, leptin resistance refers to a condition in which the body is resistant to the effects of the hormone leptin. When you have eaten enough, increased leptin levels set off a chain reaction of neuronal circuits via the hypothalamus to signal satiety and suppress appetite. These processes aim to defend your biologically determined happy weight. Supposedly, the hypothalamus of someone who is leptin resistant does not respond properly to leptin signaling. In all my research on leptin resistance, there wasn't a single study that didn't discuss the condition in relation to obesity. The claims made in these articles are rooted in fatphobia, positing that people with more fat tissue and therefore higher levels of circulating leptin do not respond "normally" to leptin signaling. The underlying message, of course, is that people in larger bodies shouldn't be as hungry because their body already has "enough" fat stores.

As someone who thinks with the utmost logic and stops at nothing to find reasons for unexplained occurrences, I determined that vague conclusions just don't cut it, such as those indicating that "a better understanding of leptin mechanisms are necessary to facilitate the development of drugs able to normalize leptin signaling with the ultimate aim of body weight reduction."[7] Perhaps, the emphasis on weight loss is the very reason scientists have not found a "cure" for leptin resistance in the first place. In point of fact, the body does not act without reason. You wouldn't have mental hunger if your body didn't need to find alternative ways to seek out food. You wouldn't be tired if you didn't need to rest. And you wouldn't be reading this book about how to bEAT extreme hunger if you didn't already believe you have what it takes. Similarly, the body does not store additional fat if it doesn't need to.

You've most likely heard the phrase "diets don't work." That's because dieting (restriction) is perceived by the body as stress. To bring itself back to safety and achieve homeostasis, the body will compensate for the restriction. When anyone tries to lose weight without proper guidance and attunement to their unique needs, the body believes there is a famine. It does not matter how many fat stores you already have, your primal brain still receives messages that your environment is not safe. In an effort to maximize your chances of survival, the body will start to conserve energy. Your ghrelin levels increase and leptin levels decrease. This perceived starvation is no hormonal problem, merely an evolutionary adaptation.

Using sheer willpower and discipline to try to lose weight does not work because it's not sustainable. Humans are wired to engage in activities that are rewarding, so setting yourself up for constant punishment and dread will inevitably lead to a breaking point. This is why the infamous "post-diet binge" is so common; after all the restriction and overexercise you've engaged in (no matter your body size), your body will become exhausted and seek compensation at some point. Bingeing on high-calorie, highly palatable foods is therefore one of the most adaptive evolutionary mechanisms, as it services two neglected needs: energy intake and a dopamine hit.

The post-diet binge usually triggers feelings of guilt and shame, causing an individual to believe they need to "get back on track" by dieting and exercising even harder. But what did our good friend Sir Isaac Newton teach us back in chapter 7? *For every action, there is an equal and opposite reaction.* Pushing your body even harder will just lead to an even harder pushback. So while one may initially lose weight through restrictive and dreaded measures, they will likely gain it back as the body aims to rescue itself.

Medically known as weight cycling and more commonly known as the yo-yo effect, the phenomenon of continually losing weight only to gain it all back (and more) has well-founded biological roots. As discussed in chapter 22, everybody has a set-point weight range, i.e., the weight range your body will naturally settle in when you are in energy balance. When you diet and fall below this range, your body thinks, "Uh-oh! We're in danger!" and will do everything in its power to bring you back into that range. The more you push your body to drop below its natural range, the more traumatized your body becomes and thus, the more likely it is to trigger mechanisms to prevent you from falling below that range again. One of these mechanisms is weight overshooting, or gaining back more weight than you initially lost.

Just as with bingeing after restriction, gaining weight after "successfully" losing it can result in feeling like a failure. You may wonder why losing weight works for everyone else but has only proven how broken your body is. You may think, "If I just had more willpower and discipline, dieting and keeping off the weight would work for me too!" So you try all the latest tips, tricks, and hacks, only to "fall off the wagon" again, confirming your belief of being a failure. Quickly, you become trapped in a cycle of dieting, weight loss, bingeing, weight gain, and a constantly looming storm cloud of negative emotions. Being in this place can cause despair and, for many, will lead to seeking external answers in ideas such as leptin resistance. Just like when I deemed my extreme hunger "invalid" because I was at the highest weight I'd ever been, you may believe you've damaged your body beyond repair. However, the complete opposite is true! The fact that your body is doing everything in its power to rescue you through weight gain and build a safety net through weight overshoot proves how well it's doing its job. When you stop messing with the natural processes and trust that it will take care of itself, your hormones will reach normal levels and you will find satisfaction.

I am fully aware that I am writing this book as someone with thin privilege, meaning I am an individual with a set-point weight range that fits society's standards for what is "acceptable." I obviously can never know firsthand what it feels like to have an eating disorder as someone in a larger body; I can only imagine that society's invalidation of your struggles and tendency to attribute them to biological or behavioral "problems" is not only discouraging but damaging. The research on how the body is "supposed" to work is heavily founded on the norms of a non-inclusive, fatphobic society, evident in articles such as those discussing leptin resistance.

Explaining the leptin mechanism and then claiming that mechanism to be broken in "obese" people is not only morally incorrect but scientifically unfounded. First, being "obese" is based on BMI, which you've already learned is complete bullshit. Second, someone's weight does not rely exclusively on the functioning of leptin (or ghrelin for that matter). Food intake and energy regulation are complex mechanisms that no amount of scientific research can ever comprehend, meaning there's absolutely no way to attribute fat storage to a single hormone. In addition, people's eating behaviors and lifestyle habits are dependent on several factors, including their genetics, occupation, income, culture, relationships, and whether or not they have a (history of) mental or physical illness – just to name a few. Similar to how no one attributes someone being in a smaller body to having "ghrelin resistance," it's about time society stopped condemning people in larger bodies to have "leptin resistance."

But what if you really are at a weight that's much higher than your set point, so much so that it poses potential health risks? Although I fully support Health at Every Size, it is important to note that this does not mean *every* body is healthy at *every* size. We all naturally have upper and lower limits within which our body functions best, and there is no denying that going drastically beyond either end of your unique weight spectrum can pose serious health consequences. Maybe you have never gone on a diet, yet your body naturally tends to put on a lot more body fat than what is accepted in today's society. Is there a reason for this? Decades of research illustrate how the genetic predisposition to store large amounts of fat can be seen as an evolutionary adaptation to facilitate survival during times of famine.

Evolutionary Adaptations to Famine

When it comes to hypotheses about evolutionary adaptations to famines, chances are you've heard of the adapted to flee famine hypothesis (AFFH). This theory by clinical psychologist and evolutionary biologist Dr. Shan Guisinger proposes that the behaviors exhibited in individuals with anorexia nervosa (AN) (i.e., restricting food, hyperactivity, and denial of starvation) are adaptive mechanisms that once facilitated migration in response to local famine.[8] Thousands of years ago, food was not as readily available as it is today. Our earliest ancestors were hunter-gatherers who relied on their direct environment for fuel. If local resources were scarce, individuals would have done better by hunting and gathering somewhere else. To migrate efficiently, individuals' bodies would have to turn off the usual adaptations to starvation, such as extreme fatigue and painful hunger pangs.

Whereas the AFFH revolutionized my understanding of anorexia and makes sense for individuals in lower weight classes, it obviously does not explain alternative responses to famine. One plausible explanation lies in the idea that famine has not been a pervasive feature of our entire history, but rather a phenomenon linked to the development of agriculture.[9] During the Neolithic era (ca. 10,000–2,000 BC), ancient humans transitioned from hunter-gatherer lifestyles to a more settled one in which they began farming and domesticating animals. While this shift had many advantages – including the ability to engage in other activities besides solely seeking food – relying on one establishment posed a heightened threat for the possibility of food shortage. If the harvest failed, members of the population that had abundant fat stores were better equipped to survive the period of scarcity.

Even though the discovery of agriculture was a revolutionary breakthrough, food supplies at the time were not as abundant as they are in our current society of mass-production. Because of this, famines were likely frequent, meaning the ability to maintain a level of additional weight remained a selective advantage. Natural selection, an evolutionary process whereby organisms that are more adapted to their environment are more likely to survive, passed their genes on to facilitate the survival of their kin to come. The adaptive, fat-storing mutations as a result of the agricultural revolution would not have had a chance to spread through the entire population in the relatively short time scale since the start of the Neolithic era, which may factor into understanding why modern society has such diversity in body size. So, if you are someone who has inherited genes that lead you to be bigger-boned and perhaps put on weight more easily than that one friend who can seemingly eat whatever they want without gaining weight, stop beating yourself up. This characteristic is part of your genetic makeup, one you literally can't change! Trying to fit society's mold of what you're "supposed" to look like is impossible, meaning that chasing this ideal will continue causing you harm. In fact, knowing what you know now about dieting and weight gain, signaling famine to your body only increases the likelihood that you will to store additional fat due to the activation of the genes that saved your ancestors.

Obviously, the opposing viewpoints presented here – anorexia nervosa as an adaptive response to famine within hunter-gatherer populations and the ability to easily store body fat as an adaptive response within agricultural ones – are largely hypothetical and simplified, to say the least. As I've said before about how we can only ever partially understand biological mechanisms, the same goes for historical findings and concurrent research. The truth is that we humans can only ever observe or document findings from our conscious awareness, an awareness that is limited beyond words. We can only study the human body based on touchpoints we already have, and we can only study history from the present moment. Furthermore, we are often restricted in semantics and labels. I have found these linguistic limitations to consistently pose a challenge when it comes to expressing my complex critiques and questions on the topics discussed. One such conundrum arises regarding the etiology and terminology of anorexia.

The term "anorexia" stems from the Greek *an-* (ἀν-, "without") and *órexis*, (ὄρεξις, "appetite") to literally translate to "lack of appetite." "Nervosa" stems from the Latin *nervōsa* ("nervous"), making anorexia nervosa mean "nervous lack of appetite." This term first entered the literature in 1873 after Sir William Withey Gull, an English physician, read a paper on his findings of starvation behaviors in some of his patients.[10] Right from the start, the description of anorexia was fatally flawed. As anyone with (a history of) anorexia knows, we do not lack appetite! If this was truly the case, people with anorexia would not think about food 24/7. In fact, several studies have shown elevated levels of ghrelin and neuropeptide Y – two potent appetite-stimulating molecules – in patients suffering from the restrictive eating disorder.[11] But here, too, a disclaimer is required, as most of the research to date is based on measurements and reports of individuals presenting with "typical" anorexia (i.e., a thin white female teenager who has an official diagnosis of anorexia nervosa and has access to healthcare). This stigmatizing exclusivity puts a big question mark next to the biological measures of anorexia in males, members of the LGBTQ+ community, people of color, and people who don't have access to healthcare, not to mention people who are not even recognized to have a disordered relationship with food due to being in a larger body.

Based on the current definition in the *Diagnostic and Statistical Manual of Mental Disorders*, fifth edition (*DSM-5*), anorexia nervosa is diagnosed according to the following criteria:

> A. Restriction of energy intake relative to requirements, leading to a significantly low body weight in the context of age, sex, developmental trajectory, and physical health.

B. Intense fear of gaining weight or of becoming fat, or persistent behavior that interferes with weight gain, even though at a significantly low weight.

C. Disturbance in the way in which one's body weight or shape is experienced, undue influence of body weight or shape on self-evaluation.

When people in larger bodies are formally diagnosed with anorexia, it is often preceded by the label "atypical." Atypical anorexia refers to an Other Specified Feeding or Eating Disorder (OSFED) and is characterized by meeting all the diagnostic criteria for anorexia nervosa except that despite significant weight loss, the individual's weight is within or above the normal range.[12]

From the already flawed definition of "typical" anorexia nervosa, it goes without saying that the definition for "atypical" anorexia is highly inaccurate. For starters, usage of the word "atypical" implies that this eating disorder is less prevalent than "typical" anorexia, which contradicts the likely estimate that people in larger bodies presenting with restrictive eating disorders are more common than those in smaller bodies. I will refrain from using statistics here, as I believe any numbers would undermine the true frequency of people who suffer from anorexia without being severely underweight, due to medical gaslighting.

Furthermore, many of the defining criteria for anorexia nervosa do not even apply to those who have received the diagnosis (regardless of body size), including an intense fear of weight gain and body dysmorphia. I myself was diagnosed with anorexia nervosa at the age of eleven, yet at the time of this writing, I am in my twenties and still do not resonate with the label at all. Many of the individuals I have worked with share my experience of being diagnosed with this illness that never felt "right." Upon reflection and after discovering I am autistic, it has become clear to me and to many of my clients that our presentations of "anorexia" were food- and exercise-related manifestations of autism all along. Due to the underrecognition and invalidation of our neurodivergence, the core of the eating behaviors was swept under the rug and stamped with the label of an eating disorder.

Circling back to the adapted to flee famine hypothesis, which places question marks next to the etiology of anorexia in non-hunter-gatherer populations, it stands to reason that similar to autism, the label "eating disorder" could collectively be considered a spectrum disorder in and of itself – one that need not be restricted (pun intended) to stigmatizing criteria including weight or shape. The common use of the word "anorexia" is misleading and is better reserved to cases of what I consider true anorexia, as in cancer patients who lose their appetite as a result of treatment.

Of course, the entire conversation about certain terminology stirs up a soup of semantics and can easily lead us down a rabbit hole of etymology, which goes beyond the scope of this book. However, I believe awareness of these linguistic flaws is an essential aspect of understanding the danger of labels (more on this in part 8), which permits you to regain power over your own perspectives and values.

Insulin

When you hear the word "insulin," you may immediately associate it with diabetes. While insulin is definitely something people with diabetes have to deal with every day, insulin is something we all have to deal with every day! So what exactly is insulin? Insulin is a hormone made by islets – clusters of beta cells – in the pancreas that plays a crucial role in regulating blood sugar levels. When you ingest calories, your body breaks down the carbohydrates into glucose, which then enters your bloodstream. In response to the rise in blood sugar levels, the pancreas releases insulin, which transports the glucose to different parts of the body. Insulin acts as a "key" that unlocks cells, allowing glucose to enter. Once inside the cells, glucose can either be used for immediate energy needs or stored as glycogen in the liver and muscles for later use.

In the case of diabetes, the affected individual either cannot make (enough) insulin or cannot effectively use it, leading to excess glucose in the bloodstream. Type 1 diabetes is a genetic condition caused by the autoimmune response against pancreatic beta cells, making the pancreas incapable of producing sufficient insulin.[13] People are born with Type 1 diabetes, meaning it is often diagnosed earlier in life and requires lifelong insulin therapy to keep blood sugar levels in check. Type 2 diabetes, on the other hand, is developed during someone's lifetime. It occurs when the body becomes resistant to the effects of insulin or fails to produce enough insulin to keep blood sugar levels balanced. The exact causes of Type 2 diabetes are unknown and go beyond the scope of this book, but one factor seems to be insulin resistance.

As with leptin resistance, there is a lack of convincing research on insulin resistance, making it nearly impossible to draw conclusions that objectively illustrate its relationship to weight and overall health. However, enough studies demonstrate that insulin resistance does in fact exist, making it helpful to understand exactly what we are talking about when referring to it. Simply put, insulin resistance occurs when insulin's target tissues (mainly the liver, muscles, and fat)[14] don't respond properly to insulin and thus are unable to easily take up glucose from the bloodstream. In response to the high levels of circulating glucose, the pancreas makes more insulin to help the glucose enter the cells. In mild cases, this increased activity allows the pancreas to make enough insulin to overcome your cells' weakened response, and there is no cause for alarm. If your cells lose too much of their sensitivity to insulin, however, it causes elevated blood glucose levels (hyperglycemia), which, over time, can lead to Type 2 diabetes.

Now, before you jump to the conclusion that you're at "high risk" for developing Type 2 diabetes if you continue honoring your extreme hunger for all the sweets and processed foods (trust me, I know that fear all too well!), it's important to recognize that Type 2 diabetes does not have one sole cause; rather, it is a combination of factors including genetic and lifestyle factors, age, ethnicity, and other medical conditions.[15] Furthermore, having insulin resistance does not immediately put you at risk for developing diabetes. In fact, anyone can develop temporary insulin resistance!

An excellent example of temporary insulin resistance is seen in some people while pregnant. During pregnancy, the placenta produces hormones that help support the growth and development of a baby. Some of these hormones, including human placental lactogen, estrogen, and cortisol, can interfere with insulin action in the person's body, making their cells less responsive to the effects of insulin.[16] As a result, more insulin is needed to maintain normal blood sugar levels. The temporary insulin resistance that occurs during pregnancy is a physiological adaptation to supply an adequate amount of carbohydrates to the growing fetus, which uses glucose as its main energy source.[17]

Similar to a growing fetus, your body requires lots of energy to heal and repair. The reason you crave so much sugar is because it's one of the most efficient fuel sources, and your body is doing its best to get you healthy as quickly as possible! And similar to a pregnant person (ironically, since you may joke that you look pregnant while bloated), you may develop temporary insulin resistance during your extreme hunger period (I'm pretty sure I did!). However, just as this insulin resistance resolves itself when hormones realign after giving birth, your hormones will even out as you feed your body back into energy balance.

When I was experiencing extreme hunger, I remember feeling shaky, sweating, and having heart palpitations. Studies have found a correlation between such symptoms and insulin resistance, but there is no evidence suggesting that insulin resistance *causes* these bodily experiences. When reading or hearing about scientific connections of any kind, it's important to remember that correlation does not imply causation. What does seem to be a recurring factor in both insulin resistance and symptoms of anxiety – including the aforementioned shakiness, sweatiness, and irregular heart rate, as well as other symptoms such as trouble concentrating and irregular breathing – is sympathetic nervous system activation. So let's consider the impact of stress on insulin levels.

Several studies have illustrated a connection between stress and insulin resistance. Throughout history, humans have developed mechanisms to optimize chances of survival in challenging and unpredictable times. These mechanisms include the ability to withstand starvation in times of famine through energy storage, the capacity to fight off infection by a proinflammatory immune response, and the ability to cope with physical stressors using an adaptive stress response.[18] In the body, energy is stored mainly as glycogen in the liver and fat tissue, which you learned is regulated by insulin action. As the manufacturers of insulin, healthy and sufficient pancreatic beta cells are of utmost importance in regulating bodily homeostasis. Stress has been shown to have a negative impact on glucose homeostasis by modifying beta cell function through activation of inflammatory responses.[19]

Inflammatory responses are an integral part of the immune system that aim to protect the body from harmful stimuli and promote healing through activation of a wide array of complex biological processes. The immune system evolved alongside the stress response, which adapted to better equip organisms with the ability to combat invaders and promote healing. For example, when you get the flu, your immune system is responsible for fighting off the virus. Specialized immune cells detect the virus and release chemical signals called cytokines to trigger an inflammatory response, recruiting more immune cells to the infection site. Different types of immune cells – such as B-cells and T-cells – work together to eliminate the virus and build immunity against it. This adaptive response aims to prevent the virus from causing future damage, thereby supporting your survival.

Stress of any kind – including stress induced by restriction and overexercise – has been shown to induce recruitment of inflammatory cells.[20] The release of corticosteroids (hormones released through activation of the hypothalamic-pituitary-adrenal axis, more on this later) and catecholamines (hormones and neurotransmitters released through activation of the SNS) activate the recruitment of leukocytes (white blood cells that are important components of the immune system), which, in turn, can cause inflammation in pancreatic beta cells.[21] All that to say, getting your body out of energy deficit and into a state of rest and digest is critical to the production of healthy insulin-producing beta cells.

Aside from damaging beta cells, insulin resistance caused by proinflammatory cytokines and stress hormones can be viewed as an adaptive mechanism to mobilize stored energy. As mentioned previously, the ability to survive famine through energy storage has been an important element of mammalian evolution. During times of trauma, stress, and/or infection, inhibition of insulin action (insulin resistance) allows glucose to be released from the liver and fat tissue to support vital metabolic processes.[22] This "adaptive insulin resistance" is repeatedly observed in a variety of conditions associated with the fight-or-flight response, such as during fasting and other times when the body may feel threatened.[23]

In conclusion, there is nothing inherently "wrong" with insulin resistance, just as there is nothing "broken" in your body if you are experiencing what seems to be leptin resistance. The body is a highly adaptive organism that activates evolutionary mechanisms to protect itself from perceived danger. To "tone down" these mechanisms and responses and support peaceful health, prove to your body that it is not in danger!

Metabolism

When you hear the word "metabolism," you may immediately jump to the thought of it being fast or slow. In today's diet-culture-obsessed society, someone with a so-called fast metabolism is praised and considered lucky for being able to eat whatever they want without gaining weight. On the other hand, people in larger bodies are often thought to have a slow metabolism and are therefore advised to eat less. Not only do these phrases reek of fatphobia, they severely simplify the complexity of metabolism.

So then what exactly is metabolism? Metabolism refers to all of the physical and chemical processes in the body that convert or use energy to sustain life.[24] It is regulated by your nervous and endocrine systems that work in tandem to maintain homeostasis and meet the body's metabolic demands. Because metabolism is a very broad term that encompasses the entirety of the body's energetic processes, referring to someone's metabolism as being "fast" or "slow" is scientifically incorrect. A better-suited formulation would be a *metabolic rate* that is higher or lower than average. Of course, this isn't a book on language formulation, so I'm going to stop myself there – what you're here for is to learn what you can expect regarding metabolism when you honor your extreme hunger!

As I explained earlier, energy deficit has diminishing effects on all bodily systems, including metabolism. When you are in energy balance, metabolic processes are supported through complex biological mechanisms including hormonal regulation, thermogenesis (heat production), and the appropriate activation of different branches of the autonomic nervous system (as discussed in chapter 23). Interference with this balance results in undertakings that ensure energy conservation and optimize chances of survival.

For almost seven years, I was constantly cold. I remember one summer particularly well, as my dad wouldn't stop commenting on the fact that I was bundled up in a blanket as we sat on the beach in tropical weather. My body's apparent inability to keep itself warm was a characteristic that didn't stand alone. Even though I was always tired, I could never sleep. Even though I was lifeless and numb, the tenacity of my eating disorder kept me slaving away. And even though I was pushing myself through what I now clearly see was physical torture, the amount of pain I endured was far from what I felt at the time.

When I gave myself full permission to eat unconditionally, my bodily experiences flipped 180 degrees. I was confronted with recurring hot flashes, sweaty palms, and smelly armpits, and I would frequently wake up in the middle of the night practically swimming in a pool of sweat. I often joked that I was going through menopause, which was ironic considering I was an eighteen-year-old female that had never menstruated. Although these symptoms are far from glamorous, changes in body temperature are a telltale sign your body is working hard to heal.

Coming out of energy deficit and paying back energy debt requires an incredible amount of calories – and if you're unfamiliar with the history of the calorie, you may be intrigued to know it was never intended to be an obsessive measurement tool now plastered on the back of every food item imaginable. The calorie originated in studies concerning fuel efficiency for the steam engine and was defined as the quantity of heat needed to raise the temperature of 1 kg of water from 0 to 1 degree Celsius.[25] In essence, it was a way to measure the amount of energy (heat) required for the most efficient way to optimize functioning.

Although you are obviously much more complex than a steam engine, your biological nature has no secret agenda besides acquiring and using fuel in the most efficient way possible. To repair your bones and organs, not to mention rebalance your endocrine and nervous systems, your body will demand foods and drinks that contain a high number of calories. And as your cells use the consumed energy for repair work, a lot of heat is generated! Because your body needs to ensure the environment stays at the optimum temperature for further repair, it will excrete that heat in any way it can. So next time you're grossed out by how sweaty you are, give your body a pat on the back for working its metabolic magic.

One of the key organs involved in regulating metabolism is your thyroid. The thyroid is a small bow-shaped gland located in the neck, just below the Adam's apple. Iodine – an essential mineral that must be obtained through food – is critical for proper thyroid function. Specifically, your thyroid produces two main hormones from the mineral: triiodothyronine (T3), which contains three iodine atoms, and thyroxine (T4), which contains four iodine atoms.[26] T3 and T4 work together to tell your cells how much energy to use, directly influencing thermogenesis, i.e., the release of heat. Because of your thyroid hormones' innate function to regulate energy, T3 and T4 play a major role in growth, repair, and development.[27]

As with any bodily system, the thyroid will slow hormone production in times of famine. Research shows that individuals with anorexia exhibit symptoms of hypothyroidism (an underactive thyroid), including bradycardia, hypothermia, hypotension, dry skin, and reduced metabolic rate.[28] Whereas the world's leading cause of hypothyroidism, Hashimoto's disease – an autoimmune disorder that destroys thyroid cells – knows no cure, symptoms of an underactive thyroid in malnourished individuals (meaning the symptoms are caused by malnutrition without underlying thyroid dysfunction) resolve with nutritional rehabilitation.[29] In fact, as your body utilizes the abundance of energy you provide it by honoring all forms of (extreme) hunger, you will likely experience *hypermetabolism*.

As the name suggests, hypermetabolism is the phenomenon of accelerated metabolic rate. Although it shares many of the same characteristics as hyperthyroidism (an overactive thyroid), the complications of eating disorders and recovery from them is usually not rooted in thyroid issues. Therefore, it's important to separate natural metabolic adjustments from clinical syndromes. Not only is hypermetabolism a completely normal part of recovery from disordered eating, it's also commonly observed in people recovering from burns, sepsis, surgery, and other traumatic injuries.[30] Depending on the severity of the burns, studies on burn victims observed a hypermetabolic state lasting up to three years.[31] Just as individuals traumatized by fire or infection need a prolonged abundance of nutrition to heal, you – as someone who has been traumatized by restriction and overexercise – need a prolonged abundance of nutrition to bring yourself back into energy balance. I know firsthand how frustrating it can be to feel like you're literally eating 24/7; what massively helped me was reminding myself that the energy I consumed ensured my body could continue healing 24/7!

Beyond the aforementioned hot flashes and sweaty circumstances, I also remember the bizarre "energy swings" I experienced during my healing period. There were times when I raided the kitchen to be met with limitless energy, but other times when I was left in a stupor. As I tried to untangle what caused my energy to swing in one direction as opposed to the other, the only conclusion I could come up with was that my body was healing – and it was going to show that off in a myriad of unpredictable ways.

If you're autistic like me, I believe the unpredictability surrounding extreme hunger and the changes that occur alongside it is one of the most difficult parts of the process. I was having a conversation with a client once in which she said, "It's not even the eating a lot I find difficult – in fact, I love that I can finally give myself permission to eat so much! It's the not knowing exactly how much I'm going to eat or how I'm going to feel afterwards that scares me." Those feelings couldn't resonate more with my own experiences. For so long, my eating disorder provided me with a sense of safety and predictability in a world that felt utterly unsafe and unpredictable. Contrary to the stereotypical portrayal of an eating disorder as being an illness attributed to people who "think they're fat" and "want to lose weight," my eating disorder was never about weight or shape. It was an unconscious manifestation of something much deeper – something that couldn't be spelled out in words.

When I discovered I'm autistic, I was finally able to comprehend the extent to which my eating disorder acted as a mask for my overlooked, and therefore invalidated, neurodiversity. I could finally see why all the approaches to "treat" my eating disorder only made it worse, and I could finally allow myself to envision a life in which I was free from my eating disorder while simultaneously embracing the traits that had expressed themselves since childhood. Of course, my autism discovery was as much of a mindfuck moment as it was pivotal.

Discovering you're autistic can feel like hearing a song you haven't heard in years but can suddenly sing all the lyrics to because the memory was always there, stored in your brain like an old cassette tape on a dusty shelf. Except in the case of autism, that song is your entire being – a being you've tried to hide in a lockbox rather than simply leave on a shelf. Where am I going with all this? Well, experiencing extreme hunger can feel similar. Going into the kitchen to grab yet another cookie only to realize you've eaten the whole pack and now have awoken the beast for loads of other treats you hadn't even thought about up until the very moment of being out of cookies feels like unlocking something that's always been lurking but you just didn't realize how extensive it was until you finally allowed it to be there (phew, that was a mouthful!).

Mood Swings

In the same way that the discovery of your unique brain can trigger a flood of emotions, nourishing your body after a period of scarcity will set the stage for a variety of moods. As you shift from a state of malnutrition to a state of nourishment, many hormonal changes will take place. This includes the hormones regulating reproduction, hunger, fullness, stress, and metabolism, but the hormones and neurotransmitters closely linked to mental state will be affected too!

Initially, my mood soared as a result of fueling myself with the nutrients my body had been deprived of for so long. I was grateful to eat everything I craved, and I marveled at the thought of my healing body. It felt so good to rest and finally experience true satisfaction. But just as my confidence took a nosedive from the fear that I was developing leptin and insulin resistance, my mental state became an unpredictable wave of fluctuations.

As touched on in chapter 26, neurotransmitters that influence mood and behavior are broadly found in the gut. So when you start to properly nourish your body and feed your gut microbiome, this will naturally impact your mental state. Whereas it would then seem only logical to feel constant elation in a healthy body, you know as well as I do that's not the case. In fact, I and many of the people I've worked with experienced incredible dips in mood on the recovery journey. Emotional changes are a natural characteristic of life, meaning the low moments are just as much a part of the process as the high ones. After all, you can't have a rainbow without rain!

Certainly, it can be discouraging to experience heightened sadness, anxiety, and irritability when you are fighting so hard to discover a life of joy. It can bring up feelings of doubt, regret, and, perhaps, like you're doing recovery "wrong." However, accepting the unhappy feelings rather than pushing them away is the key to making peace with your mental health. As the Dalai Lama so eloquently tells us: pain is inevitable, yet suffering is optional. Parts of recovery *are* painful. But remember why you chose this path: so you can stop suffering at the mercy of an eating disorder.

Rapid mood swings, like digestive issues and the other bodily changes that come with recovering from restriction, are a result of your body recalibrating. Energy deficit provides a blanket of numbness, one that may anesthetize "negative" feelings but one that equally drowns out the possibility of true presence and joy. It's the same blanket that causes physical pain to seemingly cease, pain you only feel once you start to nutritionally rehabilitate.

Aches and Pains

Whereas I had mentally prepared myself somewhat for the digestive issues that would occur as a result of increased food intake, I could have never foreseen the extent to which I would feel physical pain in other parts of my body. When I finally felt satisfied after a feast, my back would often hurt so much that the pain would shoot up my spine and radiate into a headache. I remember experiencing horrible heartburn and would feel jolts of joint aches at the most random times. The pain that commonly makes itself known in recovery can be another one of those doubt triggers, as it definitely made me feel I was doing something wrong. *I'm eating!* I thought. *Shouldn't I be feeling better instead of worse?*

Activation of the stress response triggers the release of certain hormones including adrenaline, noradrenaline, and cortisol. Not only do these molecules prepare the body to escape danger, they suppress feelings of pain. People with eating disorders engage in life-threatening behaviors on a daily basis, behaviors that most people cannot even fathom sustaining due to their inducement of pain. The reason I and many other ED soldiers could withstand the damaging consequences of our behaviors was because our threat response increased our pain threshold.

When you eat and rest, therefore proving to your body that it is no longer in a threatening situation, the pain that was there all along can hit you like a tsunami. Disordered eating is incredibly damaging to the body, so of course this damage will make itself known once it finally gets the chance. Aches, fatigue, and other unwanted physical symptoms are commonly associated with ill health. However, during

ED recovery, this discomfort is usually a sign of improving health. Detecting the damage your body has endured is one of the earliest indications that your body feels safe enough to heal, as the adrenaline rush that suppresses pain is no longer needed. To support the healing process, you must continue to prove to your body that it is indeed safe!

Edema

Edema, or water retention, is another common occurrence in recovery from restriction. There are several factors that cause the body to hold onto water, but one of main reasons for edema during extreme hunger can be attributed to kidney function. Your kidneys are a pair of bean-shaped organs on either side of your spine, below your ribs and behind your belly. They have many important functions, including filtering waste from the bloodstream to form urine, regulating your electrolytes (such as sodium, calcium, and potassium), and hormone production.[32]

Your kidneys play a crucial role in managing your body's water balance. They do this in part through osmoregulation, a process that adjusts the concentrations of water and electrolytes to maintain homeostasis and optimize internal functions.[33] When you increase your caloric intake, your body's electrolytes will naturally shift. The rise in absorbed nutrients in the bloodstream requires increased fluid levels to maintain osmotic balance, causing your body to temporarily hold on to extra water as it uses the energy for repair work and flushes out waste.

Antidiuretic hormone (ADH, also known as vasopressin) and aldosterone are two important hormones that influence water balance through the kidneys. Whereas ADH is produced in the hypothalamus and aldosterone is produced in the adrenal glands, both hormones work on the kidneys to increase water reabsorption.[34] Based on your body's unique hormonal shifts as a result of refeeding, you may or may not hold onto water as a result of changes in ADH and aldosterone. By the same token, not everyone in recovery will experience edema – and it's not because one person is doing recovery "better" than the other but because everyone's body is different. I personally never experienced swelling other than in my abdomen and face, whereas I've spoken to clients that had swollen legs, feet, arms, and hands for weeks on end. What's important to remember is that your body will recalibrate itself in its own way, a way that must be supported by unconditional permission to eat and rest.

Puberty, Periods, and PMDD

One of the most common signs of hormonal imbalance in individuals who get periods is a lack of menses. Known as hypothalamic amenorrhea, a missing period due to stress can be traced back to imbalances of the hypothalamic-pituitary-adrenal (HPA) axis and the hypothalamic-pituitary-gonadal (HPG) axis. The HPA axis is involved in the body's response to stress, while the HPG axis is responsible for regulating reproductive hormones. The HPA and HPG endocrine axes work in a harmonious and bidirectional manner, supporting both reproductive and survival behaviors.

The HPA axis is composed of three main parts: the hypothalamus, the pituitary gland, and the adrenal glands. The hypothalamus is a small neuroendocrine structure situated just above the brain stem. It controls the release of hormones from the pituitary gland, which sits just below the hypothalamus. The pituitary gland releases hormones into the bloodstream that can reach a variety of targets. In the case of the HPA axis, hormones released from the pituitary gland travel down to the adrenal glands, located just above the kidneys.

When you experience something stressful, the hypothalamus releases corticotropin-releasing hormone (CRH), which signals the pituitary gland to secrete adrenocorticotropic hormone (ACTH). ACTH travels down to the adrenal glands, where it prompts the release of cortisol, an important hormone in your body's response to stress. The HPA axis works in conjunction with the sympathetic nervous system to adjust hormones and initiate the stress response.[35]

As you may have guessed, the HPG axis is also composed of three main parts, including the hypothalamus and the pituitary gland. In contrast to the HPA axis that involves the adrenal glands, however, the

HPG axis influences the gonads (ovaries in females and testes in males). If you have a female physiology, your HPG axis is the primary generator of the menstrual cycle, which can be divided into four distinct phases: the follicular phase, the ovulatory phase, the luteal phase, and the menstrual phase. While everyone's biology is different and the exact length of one's cycle and its phases varies, below is a brief overview of what happens during each phase.

Follicular phase (7–10 days): The hypothalamus produces gonadotropin-releasing hormone (GnRH), which stimulates the pituitary gland to produce and release follicle-stimulating hormone (FSH) and luteinizing hormone (LH). FSH and LH travel through the bloodstream to the ovaries, where they stimulate the growth and maturation of follicles (sacs that contain eggs). As the follicles mature, they begin to produce estrogen, a hormone that plays a key role in regulating the menstrual cycle.

Ovulatory phase (3–4 days): The increased estrogen levels trigger a sharp rise in luteinizing hormone from the pituitary gland, causing the release of a mature egg from a dominant follicle (ovulation).

Luteal phase (10–14 days): After ovulation, the remaining follicle cells form the corpus luteum. Along with estrogen, the corpus luteum produces progesterone, a hormone that prepares the uterus for possible pregnancy.

Menstrual phase (3–7 days): If pregnancy does not occur, the corpus luteum degenerates, and estrogen and progesterone levels drop. This drop in hormone levels causes the uterine lining to shed, resulting in menstruation.

The HPG axis works similarly in people assigned male at birth, but with different hormones. In these individuals, the hypothalamus produces GnRH, which stimulates the pituitary gland to produce and release FSH and LH. These hormones then travel to the testes, where they stimulate the production of testosterone and sperm.

The HPA and HPG axes can both affect each other unfavorably when the body does not feel safe.[36] Physical stressors (including restriction, overexercise, and bacteria/viruses) and emotional stressors (including school/work, relationships, and/or having to navigate a neurotypical world as a neurodivergent individual) are all potential culprits for a hyperactive HPA axis. When your HPA axis goes into overdrive, high levels of cortisol suppress the release of GnRH from the hypothalamus, which in turn decreases the release of FSH and LH from the pituitary gland. The result is a drop in sex hormone production, leading to loss of muscle mass, reduced body hair, and reduced sex drive in all individuals, and hypothalamic amenorrhea (HA) in individuals who get periods.

Conversely, the HPG axis can also affect the HPA axis. Both estrogen and testosterone have been shown to reduce the production and release of cortisol.[37] So, when you go into energy deficit and activate your HPA axis, your sex hormones drop, which can further elevate cortisol levels. This feedback loop can only be broken by bringing your body into a calm state, which you do by eating and resting.

If you are someone who menstruates, getting your period for the first time can be one of the most remarkable experiences…exponentially so for someone who's battled an eating disorder. As I write in my memoir *Rainbow Girl*, I was eighteen years old when Aunt Flo initially made her appearance. It was a moment I had worked so hard for, a moment that had turned my ongoing efforts into a tangible victory. But the day I got my first period was also one of the most challenging days of my entire recovery journey.

Throughout my healing process, I often used my missing period as a reason to eat and rest. Bringing back an important lesson from part 1 of this book, not having my period was a huge part of my motivation for recovery. As a female, I knew an absent menstrual cycle was dangerous – the low estrogen levels as a result of HA put you at higher risk of infertility, osteoporosis, and cardiovascular disease.[38] So, when I finally menstruated and experienced all the symptoms that typically come with it, I went into a crisis. Suddenly, my extreme hunger no longer felt valid. *I had a tangible sign I was healed! Surely I didn't need to eat more than a "normal" person now?*

Shortly after getting my first period, I started restricting again. Because this restrictive behavior was far from the extremes my eating disorder had entrapped me in, it went under the radar. I justified the comeback of my "healthy" eating with the fact that I now had my period…except the thing was, I didn't. In fact, my second period didn't come until over a year later – after months of honoring my extreme hunger.

My first period occurred a few months after I had been discharged from eating disorder treatment and was clearly in a state of weight overshoot for my specific body. I had done a lot of necessary physical healing during my time in treatment, but because I did not yet know I was autistic, it left me in a worsened mental state. I was also completely unfamiliar with the phenomenon of extreme hunger, so the eating and resting I had done up until that point felt very forced – not as if it had been initiated by my own body.

The onset of extreme hunger about a year after getting my first period was a direct repercussion of depriving my body again. It had teetered in survival mode for almost seven years, thankfully to be rescued by my decision to ask for help in 2017. When it felt safe enough, my body displayed its health with my first period. But when I stopped eating an abundance of food again, my body immediately feared the comeback of the previous famine – so it decided to introduce me to something I'd never experienced before: extreme hunger.

As anyone who's experienced extreme hunger knows, it's something you're truly powerless against. Eating so much food until you feel so stuffed that you can barely move is far from a conscious choice – it's a primitive reaction that could virtually take place in a vacuum. Whether it's physical, mental, or both, extreme hunger pulls at you until you've satisfied every ounce of its desires. After about two months of doing the tango with this invisible hunger force, I menstruated a second time. Although one might think I would have learned my lesson after reverting to restriction the first time around, I was still far from wise.

I was not surprised when I got my second period. I had eaten so much and gained weight so fast that the return of proper biological functioning was practically a given. But it was precisely for that reason – it had all happened so fast – that I turned back to my "healthy" lifestyle. The amount of "unhealthy" food I had eaten during my two months of extreme hunger terrified me and caused a loss of identity. I had built my entire ego around athleticism, controlled eating, and triumphantly coming out on the other side of an eating disorder as a "perfect patient." I was afraid that if I continued to eat an abundance of food, I would condition my brain to develop some kind of food addiction.

I've never shared this publicly, but my period remained absent until I was in the middle of writing this book – more than three years after getting my second period. After I lost weight as a result of vomiting while living in San Francisco, I was hit by extreme hunger the moment I decided to move back to the Netherlands to be with my family. From October 2022 to January 2023, I ate practically 24/7. Then in February 2023, my period returned. Since then, my monthly bleed happens like clockwork!

Although living in San Francisco – and Boston thereafter – during a financially unstable time proved to challenge me in every way possible, I believe I have that difficult time to thank for the return of my period. If it weren't for going into severe energy deficit again, I likely would have not experienced my second wave of extreme hunger when I did. And because I had drastically more self-awareness, I also believe my second extreme hunger period was a gateway to reaching a level of food freedom I never even knew was possible. In fact, it was during this time of feeling so full and nauseous after extreme hunger episodes that I sat on my bed and wrote this book! Upon reflection, it is truly amazing not only how honoring extreme hunger served me, but how my experience can now also serve you.

One of the most prominent signs that continues to show up for me shortly before my period is feeling very emotional. I remember going to see my mom because I felt lonely and wanted to talk, only to start bawling my eyes out for no reason. Although we both knew this was a telltale sign of shifting hormones, my frustration about the situation only seemed to make me more emotional.

For a majority of my life, I relied on rigid structures and routines around food and exercise to stabilize my mood. Remember that numbness blanket I talked about? A healthy body with naturally shifting hormones yanks that blanket right away! Thanks to honoring extreme hunger, my mood was often a roller coaster rather than a beeline. The start or resumption of menstruation (or hormonal shifts in individuals of any gender, for that matter) can be especially challenging for autistic people because of that unpredictability aspect.

When people go through puberty, countless changes happen – people assigned female at birth (AFAB) put on more body fat, develop breasts, and start to menstruate. People assigned male at birth (AMAB) will experience voice changes and the growth of facial hair, among other developments. Anyone in puberty may experience hormonal acne caused by fluctuations in hormones, primarily androgens. Androgens are sex hormones that play a significant role in the production of sebum, an oily substance that protects your skin from drying out. Increased levels of sex hormones contribute to increased levels of sebum, which can clog pores, resulting in acne.[39]

Many of the changes that come with puberty can be so uncomfortable for autistic people that wanting to "stay young" may be a factor for restricting in and of itself. When I was a kid, I remember telling my mom that I didn't want to grow up. I never really knew why, but looking back with the autistic lens I have now, I realize it's because I was afraid I wouldn't be able to handle the responsibilities that come with adulthood. As a female, getting a period is a massive sign of maturity, which is why I believe not having a period gave me an excuse to feel younger. Ironically, I and almost every other autistic person I've met have been told that we are "so mature" and "wise beyond our years." The awareness and insight most autistic people possess at a relatively young age is a natural outcome of having to navigate a world that wasn't built for you. It causes you to have experiences (such as eating disorders) that teach you so much about yourself, providing you with an acuity that takes most people a lifetime to acquire (if at all). Perhaps the fear of adulthood is an unconscious adaptation to protect us from unleashing the full power of our autistic brain, therefore allowing us to superficially fit into a neurotypical world…but I guess that's just my philosophical opinion!

I was speaking to a student enrolled in my course *Extremely Hungry to Completely Satisfied* about how going through extreme hunger after initial signs of puberty can almost feel like going through puberty all over again. Dealing with the cravings, weight gain, mood swings, acne, and other gender-specific changes commonly associated with the teenage years can make the whole recovery experience seem surreal. The truth is, it isn't surreal; it's miraculous! Have you ever taken a moment to think about your body's ability to heal after all the trauma it's been through? Yeah, miraculous. But I know (trust me) it can often feel like the complete opposite.

As I said in a podcast episode that I recorded right before my two-month trip to Bali in 2023, the return of my period came with an intensity that frightened me.

"It feels like I have bipolar," I said during one of my emotional crying fits with my mom. Although I hesitate to share that sentence because my very last intention is to minimize the experience of people who actually have bipolar disorder (just like how people without obsessive-compulsive disorder minimize the disorder by saying "I'm so OCD" to describe their desire for order), I choose to share it with this acknowledgment because I know I'm not alone.

In the days leading up to my period now, feelings of euphoria can turn into depression in the blink of an eye. Not only that, but the preceding week is often filled with insatiable hunger that tends to shut off as soon as I start to bleed. The toughest part of it all, though, is the not feeling like myself. And I don't just mean feeling "off" or the temporary disconnectedness we all have sometimes. When I'm about to get my period, it resembles total dissociation. It's hard to describe precisely, as I don't exactly feel present in those moments, but my best attempt at explaining the experience is this: I am aware of my body and know that I'm alive on Earth, but my brain feels like a cloud that is incapable of thinking creatively.

As a neurodivergent person who is always seeking stimulation, and therefore finds it nearly impossible to "rest and relax" in the way neurotypicals might lie down at the beach on vacation, to say the week before my period is a monthly challenge would be an understatement.

But as any neurodivergent person would do when in a difficult situation, I immersed myself in research in an attempt to understand and solve the issue.

As you learned at the beginning of this chapter, the menstrual cycle has four phases throughout which hormonal levels fluctuate. Premenstrual syndrome (PMS) refers to a group of symptoms – including mood swings, fatigue, difficulty sleeping, changes in appetite, and digestive issues – that occur before menstruation. Because the menstrual cycle is such a complex process involving many different hormones and neurotransmitters, the cause of PMS is likely a response to fluctuations throughout the month.

Several studies have found that serotonin, dopamine, acetylcholine, and other neurotransmitters involved in mood processes are directly upregulated by estrogen.[40] Of particular relevance to alternating states of happiness and depression is serotonin, often called the "feel-good" chemical due to the correlation between serotonin and an overall positive quality of life.[41] The impact of estrogen on serotonin is notable in subjects across the menopausal transition, a period characterized by drastic fluctuations in estrogen levels before overall levels drop to approximately 10% of premenopausal levels.[42] The loss of estrogen at menopause results in decreased levels of serotonin and its receptors, which helps explain the symptoms of depression, anxiety, and insomnia – states that are inextricably linked to the serotonergic system – commonly observed in postmenopausal people.[43]

Postpartum depression (PPD) is another well-known occurrence characterized by low estrogen levels.[44] During pregnancy, the levels of reproductive hormones (including estrogen and progesterone) are very high. Delivery of a baby (or multiple) causes a sharp drop in these hormones, to which sensitive individuals may respond with depressive behaviors. Whereas common knowledge about PPD accepts the role estrogen plays in mental state, most people are not aware of how closely connected the hormones are to neurotransmission – so much so that some molecules function as both hormones and neurotransmitters! Research on PPD demonstrates a reduction in the levels of multiple neurotransmitters critical to mood and behavior regulation, including serotonin.

Several studies have evaluated the reward system in people with PPD by examining neural responses to infant cues – a motivationally relevant stimulus for mothers – that sheds light on a mother's dopamine function. As expected, neuroimaging studies observed increased activation of reward centers in the brain when healthy mothers saw their own infant as compared to an unknown infant.[45] In contrast, mothers struggling with PPD were shown to have reduced responses to their own infant's joyful faces.[46] These findings yield evidence of a relationship between hormone reduction and dysregulation of the dopaminergic system.

Similar to the behavioral effects of estrogen reduction surrounding menopause and pregnancy, PMS symptoms may be attributed to the hormonal impact on neurotransmitters throughout the menstrual cycle. After ovulation, estrogen drops and stays low throughout the luteal phase. So, the fact that you may *feel* low during this time is no coincidence. Naturally, the extensive documentation of hormonal influence on neurotransmitters – neurotransmitters that play a key role in neurodivergence – led me to wonder whether neurodivergent individuals are more susceptible to PMS-like symptoms. Turns out, they are!

I've never been a religious person, but the course of my life has led me to believe that there is something beyond our conscious awareness that connects us to experiences that lead to insight and enrichment. While struggling during my luteal phase one month, I opened the Instagram app to be met by a post created by a fellow autistic ED warrior and friend titled "Autism & PMDD." I'm always intrigued by new terminology surrounding autism, so of course I wanted to learn more!

PMDD stands for premenstrual dysphoric disorder and is considered to be a much more severe form of premenstrual syndrome. Individuals with PMDD may experience a wide range of symptoms during the luteal phase of their cycle. These symptoms are similar to the aforementioned mood swings, fatigue, difficulty sleeping, changes in appetite, and digestive issues commonly seen in PMS but, you guessed it, are much more extreme. In fact, unlike PMS, PMDD is an official disorder in the *DSM-5* categorized under "depressive disorders." To meet the criteria for PMDD, you must experience a total of five specific symptoms, at least one of which must be from the following group:

- feeling very irritable or angry
- feeling very down or depressed
- feeling very anxious, stressed, or tense
- avoiding your usual activities

Any one (or more) of these additional symptoms must be present (for a combined total of five symptoms) to confirm PMDD:

- difficulty concentrating
- feeling tired and very low in energy level
- binge eating or having really strong specific food cravings
- sleeping too much or having trouble falling asleep
- feeling overwhelmed or out of control
- unpleasant physical symptoms, especially breast tenderness, bloating, body aches, and weight gain

In order to be diagnosed with PMDD, symptoms must be present *only* in the week or two before your period, and they must subside within a few days of starting your period as quickly as they come on.[47] This is a critical note, as the listed symptoms are also seen in other circumstances, such as when coming out of energy deficit and in other mood disorders.

During my own luteal phase, there are always a few days where I seem to completely blank out. It can be quite scary, as the numbness can overtake me from one moment to the next, rendering me incapable of engaging in activities I usually love doing. Furthermore, PMDD can cause incredible exhaustion to the point where all I want to do is sleep – and I'm not the only one! One of my clients told me that she sleeps a whopping eighteen hours each night for two to three days during her luteal phase each month.

The exact causes of PMDD are unknown, and there is unfortunately quite a lack of research on the subject. However, there are various explanations for why someone may experience PMDD, including genetics, trauma, and hormonal and sensory sensitivities.

Genetics: Based on family studies, twin studies, and genetic studies, PMDD is thought to have a heritability range of 30%–80%.[48] Researchers have found associated variations of specific estrogen and serotonin receptor genes in individuals with PMDD compared to control subjects.[49] These findings establish a biological basis for PMDD, validating the experience of PMDD warriors and therefore paving the path to appropriate management of the disorder.

Trauma: Significant stress and trauma exposure have been associated with PMDD.[50] There are several explanations for this risk factor in and of itself, one being the tightly linked HPG and HPA axes. Furthermore, patients with a genetic predisposition for PMDD may be more vulnerable to develop PTSD in the first place due to a heightened trauma response.

Sensitivities: While I researched PMDD, the topic of hormonal and sensory sensitivities naturally intrigued me due to the associations with neurodiversity. In fact, the presence of a neurodivergent brain could rule out the need to search for different causes of PMDD altogether, considering neurodivergence is genetic and neurodivergent people are more likely to experience abuse. Furthermore, it is well established that neurodivergent individuals process sensory stimuli differently – including hormonal stimuli. That being said, let's give neurodiversity the spotlight it deserves and delve into just why neurodivergent individuals are more likely to experience PMDD.

Among the population of individuals who menstruate, current estimates show a 20%–40% prevalence of PMS, while 2%–8% experience PMDD.[51] When it comes to statistics, many people without access to healthcare are not included. Therefore, it's important to take these numbers with a large grain of salt and use them to get a general idea of the true statistics. The reason I choose to share these numbers here is because of their strong clash with the data found in the neurodivergent population. With the ongoing stigmas surrounding neurodiversity and the massive underrecognition, invalidation, and misdiagnosis of mental health conditions, it's safe to say reliable studies on neurodiversity are few and far between. However, results from the studies that *have* been conducted show significant elevation of PMDD occurrence among the autistic and ADHD population.

One study from 2008 compared 26 women diagnosed with autism with 36 neurotypical control women. The results were quite astounding: 92% of the autistic women met the diagnostic criteria for PMDD, compared to a mere 11% in the control group.[52] Another 2021 study assessing the prevalence of PMDD in those with ADHD recruited 209 ADHD women and 1,405 neurotypical controls to complete questionnaires measuring PMDD symptoms. The results indicated a 46% prevalence of PMDD in the ADHD'ers as compared to a 28% prevalence in the control group.[53] The wide 11%–28% range of PMDD found in neurotypicals begs the question of how reliable the observed 92% and 46% prevalences of PMDD in autistic and ADHD people truly are – not to mention the fact that both studies did not include AFAB individuals who do not necessarily identify as women. Yet one conclusion can be drawn: autistic and ADHD people are much more likely to have PMDD. But why?

As previously established, genetics are a proven factor for both neurodivergence and PMDD. This led me to wonder whether the genes involved in PMDD are associated with autism and/or ADHD. While the genetic research on PMDD and neurodiversity (separately and together) is relatively new, emerging studies have confirmed alterations in the expression of estrogen and serotonin receptor genes (the same genes that have been associated with PMDD) in autistic individuals.[54] Although the research on estrogen receptor genes in ADHD is limited, there seems to be a correlation between serotonin receptor genes and ADHD.[55] Speaking of which, ADHD is often associated with the neurotransmitter dopamine. However, just like in autism, research has shown serotonin also plays a significant role.

An abundance of science shows that autistic individuals have altered levels of serotonin and dopamine in the brain.[56] Whereas this fact is generally accepted within the autistic space, less is known about the role of serotonin in ADHD. Studies from animal models of ADHD indicate an intimate interplay between serotonergic and dopaminergic neurotransmission, meaning the root causes of ADHD may lie deeper than the common belief that someone with ADHD simply "lacks dopamine."[57] Because any type of neurodivergence – beyond just autism and ADHD – is genetic and expresses itself differently in each individual, it goes without saying that physiological underpinnings are infinitely variable. This genetic variance explains why not everyone who is neurodivergent has PMDD, develops an eating disorder, or becomes a victim of abuse. Overlapping scientific findings teach us a lot, but as I mentioned in my philosophical spiel in the "Evolutionary Adaptations to Famine" section, research can only be conducted based off what we already know…and as Aristotle famously wrote, "The more you know, you more you know you don't know."

While there's a lot we don't know, new research is thankfully emerging every day. One study found that individuals with PMDD have an alteration in a specific gene complex that regulates cellular response to estrogen and progesterone.[58] In simple terms, there is genetic evidence for why people with PMDD have an increased sensitivity to their reproductive hormones during the luteal phase. When paired with knowledge of neurodiversity, this is a revolutionary finding! As you learned, hormones are closely tied to neurotransmitters. This means that divergent reactions to reproductive hormones are directly linked to variations in brain chemicals and neurologic pathways that control your mood and support a sense of well-being. Because autistic and ADHD individuals already have unique levels of these neurotransmitters, we may be more sensitive to hormone fluctuations and, thus, the symptoms they bring about.

Now, you may be wondering, why spend so much time discussing PMDD and its links to neurodiversity in a book about extreme hunger? First of all, just as I learned I'm autistic thanks to recovery from an eating disorder, I discovered I have PMDD thanks to honoring extreme hunger. PMDD is something I never knew existed before my extreme hunger journey, so there's no way I could have expected to experience it! But as I promised earlier, I'm holding nothing back. I wrote this book to share my own story and research so you know what to expect, allowing you to better understand and prepare for the challenges that may come your way. As we talked about in part 1, fear is the absence of knowledge. My hope is to pave a path of breadcrumbs containing that knowledge so you can follow through with exactly what you came here to do: find freedom!

You'll notice I didn't mention bEATing extreme hunger as your reason for being here – and that's because it *isn't* the main reason. The purpose of embarking on the journey to overcoming extreme hunger is part of a much larger purpose: being able to choose how you spend your time. Dieting, disordered eating, compulsive movement – these are all behaviors that steal your time, literally making life pass you by. Since time is the only finite resource during your lifespan, don't you think it's worth spending it in a way that's truly meaningful?

Committing to recovery from my eating disorder wasn't sheerly an act of "wanting to recover" – I didn't even know what recovered meant! For me, committing to recovery was a trust fall into the possibility of a life in which I was behind the steering wheel rather than having time-consuming compulsions drive my every decision. But even committing to recovery wasn't really committing to recovery; recovery is a state, a phase between sick and recovered. And I didn't want to forever be stuck between the two. I wanted to make it to the other side, a side I'd heard other people speak of before. A side I knew in my heart and soul existed for me, too. Just as recovery is a means to an end – becoming recovered – bEATing extreme hunger is a stepping stone to a life of peace and fulfillment. Constantly thinking about food, exercise, and weight don't fit into that life, which is why taking action to prove abundance and practice acceptance are critical elements of unlocking your full potential.

Speaking of unlocking your full potential, how can you do so if you have PMDD? Although PMDD has genetic roots and is more prevalent among the neurodivergent population, this does not mean you are doomed to suffer. I truly believe all challenges we encounter in life make us stronger. When you are faced with a problem, you must think creatively and act differently, triggering the firing of new neural networks in the brain. The firing of these circuits is what creates flexibility, as your brain becomes poised for future encounters. One of the reasons gymnasts can easily do a split is because they've practiced over and over and over again, so many times that their body will one day perceive the movement as second nature. But as any non-gymnast knows, performing a split is not easy if it's your first time! Stretching of any kind can be painful, making the act of doing so seem like a challenge…because ultimately, that's all a challenge really is: something you aren't comfortable doing. Why is it uncomfortable? Because you haven't sufficiently practiced it. So how do we overcome these challenges, let alone become stronger because of them? We take responsibility for our actions.

Developing an eating disorder was not my fault, nor is anything unfavorable that happened in your life your fault. Being born into a world that wasn't built for me wasn't my fault, nor is it yours if you're also neurodivergent or disabled. Having the genetic predisposition for PMDD isn't my fault, nor is it yours if you're in the same boat. But as I've alluded to multiple times in this book, playing the blame game is never productive. It puts you in a state of victimhood, which imprisons you to a life of limitation and fear. Taking responsibility means accepting your circumstances in their entirety and choosing to make the best of them – turning lemons into lemonade, if you will!

Choosing to give up the safety and familiarity of my eating disorder challenged me because it meant I was going to take actions I had never taken before. It was scary as shit and hard as hell, but I will forever believe that my eating disorder was one of the greatest gifts I could have ever been given. The resiliency I gained through literally fighting for my life is a trait only a life-threatening circumstance could have brought on, a circumstance I attribute many of my current achievements and victories to.

As I type these words, I'm going into my last week of a two-month trip to Bali. The number of times someone's told me, "Wow! You're here all by yourself? That's so brave!" is more than I can count on two hands. People find it strange, fascinating, and impressive. But to me, it feels like second nature. I wanted to come to Bali by myself because I've accomplished so many feats independently: flying across the ocean to get help for my eating disorder, flying halfway across the world to live in San Francisco, building a business, and writing and self-publishing multiple books. To me, doing things alone is my most tried-and-true method of getting things done. Of course, I've had loads of help and wouldn't be where I am today without the support of some of the most amazing people on Earth, but when it comes to learning, my zone of genius can only fully activate in my own time and space. In fact, it's in that very time and space that I learned to optimize my biology as a PMDD'er.

If you're someone with a female physiology, you may have heard of "cycle syncing," a term coined by Alisa Vitti in her book *WomanCode*. Cycle syncing refers to a method that aligns your exercise, nutrition, and overall lifestyle with the four phases of the menstrual cycle. Along with your circadian rhythm – a twenty-four-hour internal clock that regulates your sleep-wake cycle – individuals with a female biology possess an infradian rhythm. In chronobiology (a field of biology that examines timing processes), an infradian rhythm refers to a rhythm that occurs over a time span longer than twenty-four hours. Examples of infradian rhythms include migration, hibernation, and of course, menstruation. While my eyes were opened to the idea of tapping into my uniquely female infradian rhythm and the idea of harnessing your hormones to support yourself during each phase, I found the cycle-syncing method as it's spelled out in the book quite diet-culture-y. To elaborate, Vitti includes many phrases such as "staving off sugar cravings" and puts a lot of emphasis on consuming "fresh" and "light" foods. Moreover, the provision of restrictive meal plans, food guidelines, and the mention of calories and recommending the "best" time to consume certain amounts can be really harmful to people who have spent enough of their life preoccupied with food. Perhaps most importantly, however, following the cycle-syncing method as it's advised per phase causes me to feel even more out of touch with my body than if I trust my intuition, which obviously defeats the whole purpose! To clarify, I am by no means depreciating Vitti's work, as the countless women she's helped with her methodology and approach is a true testimony to her impact. What I'm getting at is that no method will ever be one-size-fits-all.

Just as the prescriptive food and exercise advice synonymous with the cycle-syncing method may be more damaging than helpful to people who are prone to disordered eating, the idea of tailoring your life to each phase of your cycle may be counterproductive to individuals who are neurodivergent and have different gene complexes than the typical female body. Not to mention, one doesn't even have to open the book *WomanCode* to discern its lack of gender inclusivity. Although I identify as a woman, my biology does not align with the cycle-syncing method. For starters, the idea of planning exactly how I'm going to eat and move for however many days that I'm in a certain phase of my cycle riddles me with anxiety. I have established so many routines over the years that, as any autistic person or carer of one knows, are a force not to be reckoned with! Whereas my life naturally differs from day to day, I have quite a set daily ritual. Any kind of pressure to change that would massively mess with my sanity! And I don't just think that. Before I even knew my PMDD had a name, I tried the cycle-syncing method.

After reading Vitti's book, I drew the conclusion that I was merely at the mercy of really bad PMS. *If I just follow all the recommendations in this book, I'll get rid of the PMS!* I thought. But the complete opposite happened. Instead of reducing the out-of-touchness I usually experienced for the few days leading up to my period, I felt disoriented the entire month. Thinking I just needed to get used to this new approach, I continued for a second cycle. And a third. But each time, I felt worse. Not so much in a purely mental or physical sense, but instinctively. The whole pursuit didn't *feel* right. Knowing what I know now about my likely altered gene complex and sensitivities to my hormonal fluctuations, the misalignment of my feelings with "what the book says" falls into place. My motivation, energy, and aptitude for comradery clash with Vitti's explanations of how someone with a female physiology is "supposed" to feel during each phase, which led me to conclude that my divergent biology is responsible for an altered manifestation of my entire cycle – beyond the luteal phase.

Before accepting that the typical approach to cycle-syncing doesn't work for me, I thought I was the problem. Similar to how I believed my body was broken when I experienced extreme hunger while being "weight restored," I believed my years of disordered eating had damaged by body in such a way that my biological clock would forever be wrong. However, clinging to these beliefs only led me down a further spiral of victimhood. When you're trapped, you delude yourself into believing that you'll never be at your best. Because of all the work I'd done throughout my ED recovery, I knew my circumstances could always be better as long as I wanted them to be. And because I wanted to make peace with my body on a holistic level, I began to embrace my unique makeup. In doing so, I've finally learned to align my energy with my body, regardless of what anyone else is doing.

Your body (or your entire self, for that matter) is never the problem. The *problem* is the problem, and luckily real problems can be solved. In the end, a problem is nothing more than an occurrence that does not match your expectation of what you *believe* will happen. To give a tangible example completely unrelated to food or exercise, say you ordered a table. A rectangular white kitchen table, to be precise. But instead of a white table being delivered, you received a black table – ugh, now you have a problem! But is it *really* a problem? You still have your table, it's just a different color. In fact, if you had originally ordered a black table, there wouldn't even be a problem! So what's the real reason for the problem if it isn't actually the table itself? In this example, it's that you believed you would receive a white table but got a black one instead. Because the reality of the situation clashes with the belief you held, your brain has translated the situation into a problematic one – that can only be solved once you align the reality of the situation with your expected outcome.

So often, we spend our lives saving up to buy the different color table just because it looks nice in someone else's home, without appreciating the beauty of the table we already have. But we forget that we could never live someone else's life because we're not someone else! Jumping off that point, I believe a much more fitting term for a methodology that's all about supporting your hormones to optimize your body and mind is *aligning your energy*. Everyone's energy – both their supply and demand as well as in the metaphysical sense – is so drastically different that the creation of a simple method to "perfect your cycle" really is too good to be true. It doesn't account for a multitude of factors that may influence someone's infradian rhythm, including genetics, vulnerability to trauma, and neurodivergent sensitivities, not to mention gender identity.

If you're reading this as an autistic person or a carer of one, you may resonate with living in a constant state of fight-or-flight mode. The reality of being born into a world that wasn't built for you is that you are quite literally surviving in threatening circumstances. As you learned previously, perceived danger of any kind triggers the sympathetic nervous system and activates the HPA axis, which directly impacts the HPG axis. This feedback loop undoubtedly plays a role in the neurodivergent susceptibility to PMDD. Indeed, there is scientific evidence of HPA axis dysregulation in autistic individuals as well as those with PMDD.[59] Knowledge of your unique makeup and response to stress is a key part of aligning your energy, as it gives you the power to align your expectations with your realities throughout your cycle.

As a neurodivergent business owner, my to-do list is never-ending. Most days are packed with activities that require lots of set-shifting (also known as task-switching), which has my mind regularly racing. Although this may seem like I'd constantly be overstimulated and unable to function, I wouldn't want it any other way! I am so passionate about the work I do, which is why my love for Liv Label Free (almost) always prevails over the frequent bouts of overwhelm and fear. Aside from the physical discomfort and raging return of extreme hunger during my monthly "PMDD week," my brain's transformation into a dissociated cloud is the most difficult part. No matter how much I want to, my mind seems to be incapable of forming any kind of comprehensive thoughts. This makes content creation, coaching, and almost all the other tasks within my business nearly impossible to execute.

Knowing my energy will be unaligned with the pursuit of my work that week, I am able to align my expectations with each month's upcoming reality. Instead of keeping my schedule the same and forcing myself through the misery of attempting to work, I keep that week completely open – no appointments, no writing goals, no pressure. What used to be a time of fear and feeling like a failure has turned into a phase of rest and rejuvenation, one that has inevitably contributed to feeling like a power-woman when my motivation is back! To return to the idea that a problem is nothing more than an unexpected outcome, my PMDD is now also no longer a problem – it's a part of my life I've accepted and adapted to. So, if you struggle with "period problems" of any kind, ask yourself: What changes can you make in your life to align your energy? How can you alter your expectations throughout your cycle? Living in harmony with your biology will be a surefire shift from how you may have been approaching life for however long you've been on this planet, but remember that change brings about growth, and growth is the foundation of strength.

Sleep

Now that we've touched on the hormonal changes that may impact your infradian rhythm, it's time to talk about what you can expect when it comes to your circadian rhythm. Your sleep-wake cycle is guided by a delicate dance of hormones that must be functioning properly to fulfill your sleep needs. Melatonin, often referred to as the "sleep hormone," may come to mind when conjuring up a connection between hormones and sleep. But as with all internal systems, the process of sleep is much more complex than the working of a single hormone.

If you ask my parents about my sleeping habits as a kid, they'll be quick to tell you, "She never wanted to sleep!" I would spend hours crying in my crib until my mom or dad would surrender and cradle me to comfort. They would softly sing until my eyes shut, then carefully place me back in my baby bed. Sometimes, this worked. More often than not, my hypersensitivity to their detachment would leave me crying all over again. Although I thankfully (for them) stopped crying as I grew older, I remember making up excuses to stay up late for as long as I can remember. Some of these were utterly ridiculous, including my claim that "going to bed later helps me wake up earlier." As a very logical person, I will forever wonder what part of my brain that claim came from!

Another seemingly illogical piece of my sleep puzzle is that my lack of desire for sleep never seemed to match my true need for it. I may have had difficulty shifting from wakefulness to sleep mode, but once I eventually fell asleep, I practically transformed into Sleeping Beauty! I have always required more sleep than my peers, which I believe is attributed to the overactive autistic brain. At the time of writing this book, I know I function optimally when I get nine to ten hours of sleep a night. Do note my word choice here: *optimally*. Just because I know I need that much sleep doesn't mean I always get it. I still struggle with unexpected insomnia, especially during my PMDD week. Sometimes, I'll wake up in the wee hours of the morning, exhausted yet unable to transform from a state of wakefulness to a state of sleep. Suffice to say, sleeping has never been my forte – which appears to be a common occurrence among the autistic population.

While it's hard to imagine that my sleeping issues could get any worse, my eating disorder succeeded at the herculean task. However, when looked at through a biological lens, the impact of disordered eating on sleep may not be so confounding after all. When you go into energy deficit, your brain perceives a famine. Because food shortage is one of the biggest threats to human survival, a variety of bodily mechanisms are triggered to bring you to safety – including activation of your sympathetic nervous system (SNS) and the hypothalamic-pituitary-adrenal (HPA) axis. As you learned previously, your SNS is the division of the autonomic nervous system responsible for the fight-or-flight response, while your HPA axis is the hormonal pathway that responds to stress through the release of cortisol. Predictably, initiation of the body's stress response results in insomnia, since sleeping is your body's last priority if you need to escape danger. Circling back to autism and living in what seems to be a constant state of fight-or-flight mode, sleep difficulties within the neurodivergent population are no longer puzzling. In the context of malnourishment, a constant state of hyperalertness would heighten your chances of acquiring food, which is closely linked to the hunger and fullness hormones discussed earlier.

When you are not eating enough, your ghrelin levels rise to promote food-seeking behavior. Sleeping would drastically reduce the allotted time for this, which is why insomnia may be considered a natural adaptation to obtain fuel in scarce circumstances. On the other hand, leptin levels are a direct reflection of body fat percentage and inhibit the release of certain neuropeptides, including neuropeptide Y. When you do not have adequate levels of body fat, lack of leptin prevents the signaling of satisfaction. And if your body does not feel satisfied (and therefore, does not feel safe), you will be held back from the opportunity to slip into slumber. After all, natural selection would have made a grave mistake if it promoted sleep (a time of growth and restoration) when there was not enough available energy to support these recuperative processes!

Although many of my eating disorder years are a blur, I have several memories that are as vivid as physical pictures. One particular snapshot takes place on a night when I was fourteen. It was around 1:00 a.m. and I had been tossing and turning in my bed for hours, unable to mute the thought of devouring a twelve-count box of chocolate-coconut granola bars in one go. I would play the potential scene in my head over and over again, filling in every detail from tiptoeing down the stairs into the kitchen to opening the cabinet that contained the granola bars. Somehow, I made it to the morning without turning my fantasy into a reality, only to "give in" to my craving by taking one single bar to school the next day. It's reflecting on moments like these that I struggle to fathom how I was able to resist my ever-present mental hunger for such a long time. What's more, moments like these shed light on how "normal" it actually was for me to eat the amount of food I did during my period of extreme hunger – nearly five years after the chocolate-coconut granola bar reverie.

Throughout my years of disordered eating, I experienced many nights that were physically sleepless and mentally food-full. I would visualize all of the foods I was restricting, almost tasting the plenty through the extent of my imagination. Obviously, I managed to drift off at times, but the nightmares about bingeing seemed to make insomnia the more favorable option. One night, I woke up in a panic, sweating and shaking out of fear that my nightmare had been real life. I had eaten an entire 1 kg (2.2 pound) bag of *pepernoten*, Dutch spice cookies comparable to mini gingersnaps. The vision had felt so real that I felt physically sick, sending me into a semiconscious daze that didn't end until I was hit by a wave of relief in the morning.

In an attempt to drown out both the insomnia and the nightmares, I researched sleep supplements – after all, my belief at the time was that supplements would fix everything. I started taking melatonin, what most people know as an over-the-counter sleep aid. What I didn't yet know was how melatonin is naturally produced in the body and what impact stress has on its function.

Melatonin is a hormone produced by your brain in response to darkness, and it plays a key role in your body's 24-hour clock. It's secreted by the pineal gland, a small endocrine gland located in the center of your brain. The pineal gland receives input about the state of the light-dark cycle from the suprachiasmatic nucleus (SCN), also known as your body's master circadian pacemaker or central biological clock.[60] The suprachiasmatic nucleus is strategically located behind the eyes, making it highly responsive to light and dark cycles. When it's light out, your SCN signals the pineal gland to inhibit melatonin production and thus promote wakefulness. When it's dark, the SCN stimulates the pineal gland to produce melatonin and induce sleep. You may have heard that being on your phone or watching TV before bed can disrupt your sleep. Although most viral "health" advice nowadays is more sickening than helpful, this happens to be true! The blue light emitted from electronic devices inhibits activity of the SCN, leading to reduced stimulation of the pineal gland and ultimately resulting in decreased melatonin production.

If melatonin is dependent on signaling from the pineal gland through light signals from the SCN, how can stress and malnutrition interfere with sleep? Aside from an adaptive state of wakefulness to protect you from potential danger and support food-seeking behaviors as mentioned above, hormonal and neurochemical imbalances in the body can inhibit the production of melatonin. One of these imbalances can be traced back to inadequate serotonin, which you learned is a neurotransmitter that supports positive mood. What you may not yet know is that serotonin is a precursor to melatonin, meaning it's an essential building block for melatonin's synthesis.[61] When the body believes it's time to sleep, the SCN stimulates the pineal gland to become active, giving rise to melatonin production. Through a series of enzymatic reactions, specialized cells in the pineal gland convert serotonin into melatonin, which is then released into the bloodstream. As you can conclude, lack of serotonin leads to the pineal gland's inability to produce sufficient melatonin, resulting in poorer sleep. Not only is this mechanism an explanatory factor for why neurodivergent individuals – who have altered serotonin levels – may struggle with sleep, but variations in the serotonergic system also help us decipher why malnourished individuals experience melatonin malfunction.

Serotonin is made from tryptophan, an essential amino acid. Amino acids are the basic building blocks of proteins, which are involved in virtually all biological processes. There are twenty known amino acids, of which nine are called *essential* amino acids, while the remaining eleven are called *nonessential* amino acids. Considering all amino acids are essential to life, this distinguishing terminology is questionable. Nevertheless, essential amino acids cannot be synthesized by the body, meaning they must be obtained through diet. In contrast, your body *can* produce nonessential amino acids. When you are restricting though, your body falls short of all amino acids; you're not getting sufficient essential amino acids through your diet, but your body is also unable to synthesize nonessential amino acids due to a lack of building blocks. Adequate levels of tryptophan, an essential amino acid, must be consumed in order to synthesize sufficient amounts of serotonin. Foods high in tryptophan include whole milk, bananas, cheese, nuts and seeds, bread, and chocolate.[62] Uncoincidentally, these foods tend to be the main culprits of a dieter's demonization list, making the combination of healthy serotonin levels and disordered eating behaviors an unsolvable equation. Thankfully, extreme hunger knows what's up: it causes you to crave foods that will not only bring you back into overall energy balance but also fix the hormone and neurotransmitter imbalances caused by malnutrition.

According to the science laid out in this book, the logical outcome of eating and resting is achieving energy balance and having everything in your body running like a well-oiled machine in no time. But I don't think I have to tell you that this machine will take many unexpected blows as it recovers from the time you spent maltreating it! A prime example is the all-too-familiar digestive issues that can cause you to feel your hard work is making everything worse. You also learned about several hormones that will shift and how you need to give your body time to recalibrate before throwing in the towel and giving in to the temptation of the perceived safety of disordered eating. Similarly, you will not instantly switch from battling insomnia's cruel grip to finding solace in the arms of tranquil serenity. Just as my digestive issues and hormonal shifts only seemed to bring about more troubles while I honored my constantly unpredictable extreme hunger, my sleep habits became equally iffy.

During the costly process of bodily repair, it is only natural to require extensive amounts of shut-eye. Especially after losing slumber due to insomnia, sleeping is a critical component of healing your body. I was most grateful when my sleep started improving as I ate my way out of energy deficit, but this was unfortunately not a linear path. Some nights, I would drift off in the blink of an eye, catching an uninterrupted twelve or thirteen hours of sleep. Other nights, I would toss and turn nonstop, only to become hungry and have yet another feast in the wee hours of the morning. Whereas your body's varying initiation for sleep and food can be highly frustrating, embracing it is the only way through. When you are still on the path of proving abundance to your body, it does not yet fully trust that food will always be there. Therefore, difficulty with sleep and wanting to eat in the middle of the night make complete biological sense – your body is just helping you survive! Allowing your primal instincts to take the reins and permitting yourself to eat and rest whenever your body asks for it is an essential stepping stone on the journey to freedom. When you consistently prove to your brain that food is abundant and that you can rest whenever you need, it will stop worrying about energy shortages and thus free up time and energy to reshape your life from a state of "in recovery" to fully recovered.

Even today, giving myself unconditional permission to eat and rest is an important part of my fully recovered life. As I've struggled with sleep since my youngest years and still experience unexpected restlessness from time to time, I am aware that chasing the ideal of a perfect sleep-wake cycle is as detrimental as chasing the ideal of an eating disorder's delusions. Furthermore, time changes – such as from traveling or daylight savings – will mess with even the most punctual sleepers, emphasizing that everyone grapples with sleep from time to time. A valuable question to ask yourself when bodily processes of any kind are compromised is this: What aspects of my life are posing a perceived threat? In the end, stress is like a hidden toxin that is capable of permeating every corner of your health. You can consume all the probiotics, eat all the "right" foods, and follow every health guru's advice to "balance your hormones," but if your body feels it is in danger, your digestion will be compromised and your hormones will be out of whack. Similarly, it doesn't matter how well-planned your bedtime routine is or how much calming tea you drink; if you're stressed, your primitive responses will keep you alert. Taking a holistic approach to all aspects of your life is the key to health, as ultimately, a healthy body is one whose parts work together in harmony.

PART 8

LIVING LABEL FREE

If bEATing extreme hunger is all about ruling out restriction and proving abundance, what could possibly be left? Although restriction may be the root cause of energy deficit, restriction itself has a much deeper root that must be addressed to manifest abundance. Liv Label Free establishes the root of restriction as labels. You and I both know that you didn't start restricting for the sake of restricting. Your restriction occurred for a reason (or reasons), which gave you the motivation to pursue an endeavor of limitation. Even if the restriction started out unconsciously, labels caused you to obtain limiting beliefs.

Labels are all around us. In fact, you were labeled the moment (or maybe even before) you came out of the womb! From a quick look at your genitals, a doctor labeled you either a "boy" or a "girl." Although the doctor – and society at large – may believe you *are* one or the other, gender is an illusion, a tip of the biological iceberg that is infinitely unknowable. When you attach a label to something, you believe you know what it is. However, you cannot truly know what it is, as it has unfathomable depth. The rise of individuals coming out as LGBTQ+ is a beautiful illustration of this depth, as it epitomizes the colorful nature of human existence; an existence that cannot be simplified down to the labels "male" or "female," in addition to how they are "supposed" to act. But if human existence, not to mention everything beyond it, is so impossible to grasp, why do we have labels in the first place?

When it comes to labels, it's essential to understand that they are not inherently bad – that would only create more polarization, which is exactly what the label-free philosophy empowers you to break away from. Part of my role as a guide is to help my students distinguish the intention behind their labels so they feel empowered to move in the direction of their goals rather than being held back by the limitations of their fears. That being said, there are two types of labels: labels rooted in fear and labels rooted in love.

Labels rooted in fear are labels that limit you from achieving your full potential. Because FEAR is False Evidence Appearing Real, fear-based labels convince you that something either is not possible or will lead to something horrible. A fitting example discussed throughout this book is the fear that you will never stop eating. By believing you will never stop eating, you have inherently adopted the label, and therefore the identity, of "a person that will never stop eating." As you learned in chapter 17 on junk food (another restrictive label), confirmation bias causes you to seek information that confirms your current beliefs while rejecting information that challenges them. The danger of internalizing fear-based beliefs, then, is that you create a self-fulfilling prophecy of spiralizing fear. Let's continue with the example that you will never stop eating: internalizing this belief causes you to seek validation of this truth while overlooking any alternative possibilities. Eventually, it becomes impossible to take actions that align with a life of freedom, as your unconscious mind will forever convince you that taking such actions aren't worth it. So, to open your mind – and therefore your reality – to the possibility of a life in which you will feel satisfied, you must know how to shift limiting beliefs to empowering beliefs.

In contrast to limiting beliefs that stem from fear, empowering beliefs stem from love. This is also where the upside of labels comes into play. Since humans cannot communicate via telepathy (although I guess that would be nice sometimes), we must use words and phrases to express ourselves. When you use words in a way that optimizes functionality, and therefore supports the well-being of yourself and others, you are using the power of love-based labels. Circling back to my elaboration on the terminology "extreme hunger" in chapter 5, the only reason for this nomenclature is to clarify my message and reach the people I aim to help. As I have elucidated throughout this book, "extreme hunger" isn't truly extreme; it's merely a reaction to the extreme restriction and compensation. However, using this label, while attentively bringing awareness to its context, radiates love as it helps me help you.

Another example of love-based labeling is using the word "autistic." When I speak about the Liv Label Free philosophy, I almost always get the question *Isn't autism a label?* Of course it is! But because existence is so incomprehensible, the ability to communicate through language is a true advantage. After all, it would be quite difficult to read or write if we still grunted like cavemen! Just as using the term "extreme hunger" in the title of this book helps me reach you, which in turn helps you improve your quality of life, the label "autistic" helps autistic individuals understand themselves, allowing them to improve their quality of life. Using love-based labels sets the stage for forming empowering beliefs, which are beliefs that open your mind to new and improved possibilities.

Module 1 of *Extremely Hungry to Completely Satisfied* guides you step-by-step through the process of shifting a limiting belief to an empowering belief, providing you with examples that have led to breakthroughs in hundreds of my former students. Rewiring your belief system to replace fear-based labels with love-based ones is essential to not only overcoming extreme hunger but also shedding yourself of the guilt and shame that you've been conditioned to feel in many aspects of your life. In the following chapters, we will unpack common types of limiting labels, their implications, and how shifting them paves the path to a life you love.

27

TOO MUCH IDENTIFICATION?

One of the most common forms of labeling is using the word "too." As with all labels, the word is used so unconsciously that when you first become aware of it, you'll notice how often it presents itself! Not only in your own mind and thoughts, but most conversations these days seem to revolve around the term. In fact, people rarely have face-to-face conversations anymore because they say they have too little time. Even digitally, most communication revolves around being too busy, having too little energy, work or school being too difficult.

In the eating disorder recovery space, the word "too" comes up a lot as well. *I'm eating too much. I'm gaining weight too fast. I'm craving too much junk food.* While the label "too" is a lot more nuanced than some black-and-white labels – including good/bad, right/wrong, healthy/unhealthy, etc. – I kick this section off with "too" because it's such a clear illustration of how subjective labels are. For what actually defines whether something is too [insert unwanted circumstance here]? What defines too little time, too much food, or recovery being too difficult?

Subjectivity is tightly intertwined with your identity, which is founded on your belief system. Because your beliefs cannot be felt, heard, or seen, subjective labels give you a tangible way of expressing what your conscious mind perceives as fact. Your perception of truth is based on everything you have learned – and therefore have been conditioned to believe – throughout your life. After all, no child is born with an inherent understanding of what is "right" or "wrong."

When a baby says their first "mama" or "papa," they are cheered on, conditioning them to label their parents as such. When they don't get what they want and throw a tantrum, they are scolded, conditioning them to believe that throwing a fit isn't the best way to meet their needs. As a growing child's behavior is either applauded or criticized, they develop values that influence what they believe they should and should not do – beliefs that lay the foundation for the rest of their life.

A person's identity comes to rest on this foundation. They believe they are the child of "mama" and "papa," but only because of the meaning they've been conditioned to attach to these words. After all, the names for a mother and father are merely a combination of letters, letters that happen to look and sound different based on the language in which they are being said. But can the child's so-called mama and papa really be simplified to mere letters? Is that all they are? Of course not. The words "mother," "father," "child," "friend," etc., are all ways in which communication is made possible. The child may grow up to become a writer, a runner, or even a parent themselves. When these terms are used from a place of love, that is, to improve function, everyone's life becomes easier. The danger of labels only arises when we lose our identity in them.

Your identity is formed through everything you believe you are. The word "identification" is derived from the Latin word *idem*, meaning "same," and *facere*, which means "to make." So to identify with something means to "make it the same" as you. As your identity influences your actions, an identity that is aligned with your core values provides you with a powerful force from which you can manifest your wildest dreams. For example, I identify as a writer. This identity rests on my belief that shared wisdom is one of the keys to true connection, and that through sharing my lived experience and acquired knowledge, I can help others overcome the same obstacles I once faced. Because I identify as a writer, I take actions that align with that identity…in other words, to make a writer the same as me. And what do writers do? They write.

As you learned in part 1, habits are the result of consistent action over time. Therefore, your beliefs form your identity, which forms your actions, which form your habits. As a writer, I have a daily habit of writing. It's how I feel a sense of purpose and fulfillment, for when I have written, I have quite literally fulfilled my perceived purpose. However, if it so happens that I miss a day – say I did research, had client calls, or was occupied in other ways – I don't beat myself up over it. I may be a writer, but that's not all I am. This awareness is a crucial aspect of living label free. Without being able to separate yourself from labels, your identity becomes so intertwined with those labels that you don't know who you are without them.

This loss of identity is a frequent occurrence in the world of eating disorders. When people first approach me for coaching, they often say, "I don't know who I am without my eating disorder." This may or may not resonate with you; it definitely did with me! For nearly seven years, my life revolved around servicing the needs of an eating disorder. That is, my actions, which eventually became my habits, came to rest on the belief system of the illness. Because your eating disorder is a parasite, an external identity that is not inherently *you*, you will never find fulfillment within its grasp.

Unfortunately, you have been conditioned to believe that you will find yourself beyond yourself. In other words, labels sell you on identity enrichment. Diet culture does this most prominently: "If you buy our product, you will be happy." However, you may also do it unwittingly: If I eat like that YouTuber, I will have their body. If I engross myself in recovery content and go "all in," I will be equally "in recovery" as other ED warriors. The aspiration to find happiness through ownership (such as having physical products, but also in the metaphysical sense, such as having the same diet or lifestyle as people on the internet), however, is the greatest error on the journey to discovering your true self.

Descartes said, "I think, therefore I am." Thus, the more (knowledge) you have, the more you are. But is that really so? If you have more possessions, more accomplishments, more labels, does that really change your intrinsic worth? In a sense, Descartes noted his famous line while completely trapped in his ego, unaware of his subjectivity. Because the ego – your sense of *I* – believes that *having* more equates to *being* more, it will forever want more. This persistent desire is at the root of an eating disorder's insatiable nature. Similar to a cancer cell, whose only goal is to multiply itself, an eating disorder brings about its own destruction by destroying the very organism of which it is a part. So the feeling of emptiness that comes with letting go of your eating disorder could not be more mislabeled. You are not actually empty. Rather, you are closer to being *you* because you no longer have the mask that gave you a false sense of completeness.

Because most people are unaware that true completeness is found within oneself, they continually replace one sense of identity with another. When it comes to eating disorder recovery, that label is precisely where the next entrapment happens: to be "in recovery." When my actions were governed by the belief system of my eating disorder, life was quite simple. It wasn't joyful, but it was simple. The black-and-white thinking that an eating disorder transforms into a reality lessens the overwhelm of a life you're afraid you can't handle the responsibilities of. What do I eat? *The lowest-calorie option.* When do I eat? *Only at certain times.* How should I exercise? *I just follow my daily routine.* This simplicity provides a cloak of control, as the limitation makes life seemingly overseeable. After all, overwhelm is merely the result of not having an overview.

As most people with an eating disorder do, I reached a point where I felt I could no longer live that way. That was also the moment I realized I wasn't in control – my eating disorder was controlling me. So I decided I was going to let go of my eating disorder. However, this endeavor was far from simple. If my life was no longer going to revolve around food and exercise, I believed I needed to find a replacement. But what? I had been so young when I developed my eating disorder, I had no real touchpoints of a life that was free from one. So I figured the answer would come to me while I was in recovery.

I ate more. I rested. I started sharing my story online. I changed my Instagram username more times than I can count, constantly searching for a name that would match who I believed I was. I became vegetarian, then vegan. I called myself a "foodie," then a "blogger." Although I was "weight restored" and "healthy," my health was far from restored. In fact, I experienced what most people would label as an "identity crisis."

After a few years of being stuck in what many people in the ED recovery space refer to as "quasi recovery," I decided I wasn't doing recovery "right." Eating disorder recovery was about rebelling against diet culture, allowing all foods, going out to eat, and basically doing everything opposite of what you did when your eating disorder was behind the wheel, right? So they say. Admittedly, when I decided I would recover from my eating disorder, I had only decided that because I was going to recover "the healthy way." I was going to gain weight by eating whole grains, fresh produce, and non-GMO peanut butter. I was going to go to the gym because that's what I saw all these other "recovered" influencers doing. But because fulfillment cannot be found in external circumstances, I reached a point when what seemed to work for all those what-I-eat-in-a-day and how-I-train YouTubers just left me feeling more stuck. So instead of striving for the "balanced" recovery approach, I decided I needed a new strategy. That's when I discovered "all in" recovery.

28

ALL IN RECOVERY

Similar to how the term "cycle syncing," coined by Alissa Vitti, has become a hype word among the female hormone gurus, "all in" has become a raging term in the ED recovery community. However, to be "all in" was never intended to mask the identities of eating disorder sufferers, a phenomenon all too common nowadays.

The "all in" approach is described by Nicola Rinaldi and coauthors in their book *No Period, Now What?* as a method to help recover your menstrual cycle through increasing your food intake and reducing exercise. The term "all in" refers to fully committing oneself to the healing process. Due to the strong overlap between hypothalamic amenorrhea, eating disorders, and disordered eating, along with certain influencers documenting their "all in" journeys, it's no wonder a label signifying full commitment has gained so much popularity within the eating disorder recovery space. So if full commitment is what recovery is all about, what's wrong with using the term "all in"?

There is never anything inherently "wrong" with using labels of any kind. To label any circumstance as right or wrong is another form of labeling in and of itself! The problem with the "all in" approach in the context of healing from an eating disorder, however, is that the full commitment is usually not made to oneself or discovering one's true identity. Rather, the commitment is made to *recovery*.

Letting go of an eating disorder – or, better said, the identity of one – is one of the greatest blows to the ego. Because your ego believes that having more equates to being more, the ownership of an eating disorder provides you with a falsely superior identity. The feelings of superiority that come with an eating disorder are rarely discussed, but they are in fact one of the greatest forces that keeps the eating disorder ego alive. For if you were not better or special with it, you would have let the ED go a long time ago. Of course, your true self knows an eating disorder does not make you superior but has actually led to a life that's inferior. This awareness – that is to say, observing the eating disorder from *your* perspective rather than from its subjective perspective – is the first step to separating your authentic identity from that of the eating disorder.

Unfortunately, the ego's driving force is desire. It tricks you into thinking that salvation – whether this be accomplishments, experiences, or the all-too-common "I just want to be happy" – can be found in external circumstances. People believe they need a new car or that they need to take a vacation to be happy. But if external circumstances were truly the driver of internal fulfillment, people who barely possess anything would be the unhappiest people on Earth. Yet it's these very people that seem to be the most at peace. Therefore, the illusion of joy that comes from certain acquisitions or experiences does not last for more than a mere moment, causing you to forever want and chase the next illusion.

I propose that the state of being "in recovery" – whether this be eating disorder recovery, quasi recovery, all in recovery, the Minnie Maud method, or whatever label you use to describe your state of being – is the next illusion after an eating disorder. It allows you to identify with a label that's not quite your eating disorder but equally couldn't be further from your true self.

When I first decided to go all in, I was excited. I was no longer going to identify as someone with an eating disorder! But it was at that very moment that I adopted a new identity: someone *in recovery* from an eating disorder. From the outside, it seems like this would be the logical next step. You go from identifying with an eating disorder to identifying with recovery to identifying with yourself, right? In reality, that's not quite how the cookie crumbles.

Where your attention goes, energy flows. When you attend to your eating disorder thoughts, you are providing them with energy to influence your belief system. This concept applies to recovery in the same way. When you focus all your energy on recovery and making sure you're doing it "right," you will forever stay stuck in a state of being "in recovery." Obviously, this defeats the entire purpose of recovery! Whereas the phrases "choose recovery" and "go all in" are meant to be encouraging, focusing on recovery creates the egoic illusion that recovery is the be-all and end-all. In reality, recovery is a means to an end – or rather a start – of living your life. Because isn't that your goal? To identify as yourself? To identify as someone who is free?

It wasn't going "all in" that was exciting; it was everything I associated with the *label* of going "all in" that put me on cloud nine: eating whatever and whenever I wanted, resting, living without the restrictive rules my eating disorder had confined me to for so long. But in essence, the characteristics I believed were entangled with the label "all in" weren't part of that label at all. Those characteristics are all habits of someone who identifies as free. And when you're free, you don't need a label, because you have nothing to prove.

The entire "recovery community" is filled with people who identify with certain labels. You have the vegans, the gym junkies, the foodies – hell, I know firsthand how convincing it is to believe that adhering to a certain label will save you from your eating disorder! But the danger of these labels – especially as they are portrayed on social media in such a heroic light, causing you to compare and feel you need to do the same to achieve a life of freedom – is that they are just that: labels. If someone's definition of "recovered" is founded on something external, what happens when that label is removed? Just like a house will collapse if you remove the ground underneath it, your state of being "recovered" will collapse if you remove whatever circumstance you built it on. The only thing you ever have – always – is yourself. So if you look everywhere except for within, how do you ever expect to find yourself?

This was the very realization that prompted me to become Liv Label Free. After going through countless labels – inflicted upon me by both others and myself – I learned that nothing outside of me was going to save me. Only I, or rather awareness of myself, could save me. The ego and awareness of the ego cannot exist at the same time, meaning that you must know how to zoom out before creating your life's game plan. This is where coaching, courses, and other types of guidance play a key role on the freedom journey, as a guide provides you with a perspective you are literally incapable of taking on by yourself. You can't read the label when you're inside the jar! Of course, accepting help, let alone asking for it, can be a herculean task. This has to do with the common identity role of the victim.

29

VICTIMHOOD

In her book *The Choice*, Edith Eger eloquently expresses how "many of us stay in a prison of victimhood because, subconsciously, it feels safer." You go in constant search of the "why," believing that if you can just figure out the root cause of your perceived problems, you will magically find the solution and be set free from your suffering. However, looking for what caused your circumstances provides a new level of suffering, as it keeps you trapped in the past.

Much of my time in therapy was spent looking for the supposed "traumatic experience" that had caused my eating disorder. The reasons some of my therapists came up with are utterly beyond me, one of which was that my stressful birth was the seed of an eating disorder that would lay dormant until it was ripe enough to sprout. Many of my clients have shared similarly ludicrous experiences, and we often end up laughing at our conclusion that the therapy itself was the most traumatizing experience of all! Whereas I am in no way discrediting trauma and absolutely believe it plays a role in the development of illness, looking for the "why" prevents you from taking action in the present moment. It means searching for someone or something to blame so you can become angry with whatever you find. However, that anger is negative energy that takes away from the energy you could be using to move forward.

Even if it's not a trauma, "blaming" your eating disorder on any external circumstances, whether this be genetics, undiagnosed autism, or other factors out of your control, is born from the victim mindset. The ego's constant search for more – including the search for more reasons to hold at fault – serves as a way to confirm your role as a victim, which excuses you from rolling up your sleeves and taking responsibility. It's true that genetics, trauma, and other health conditions and diagnoses can contribute to the development of an eating disorder. As I've shared many times, I believe my eating disorder was a manifestation of undiagnosed and invalidated autism. However, thinking about what "could have been" had I known I was autistic earlier on would not help me. If anything, it would precipitate feelings of regret and sadness, which would only set off a chain of more negativity. Instead, I have chosen to focus my energy on what I can do with the knowledge I now have. It's remarkable how that mindset shift has not only given me excitement for the future, it's also given me gratitude for the past. If it weren't for my eating disorder, I wouldn't be doing the work I am today. In fact, if it weren't for my eating disorder, this very book would not exist!

So how do you make peace with your past? How do you let go of the labels that have been placed upon you, whether by others or by yourself? You start by forgiving. Victimhood cannot exist without a victimizer, just as you cannot be right without making someone or something else wrong. This egoic mind pattern is the core motivation for the toxic clinician-patient relationship in which an individual is written off as "too complex" or "hopeless," an experience close to my heart and unfortunately all too common.

From the day I was kicked out of the eating disorder treatment system with the message that I "just had to accept I was never going to get better," I was angry. How could that woman have said that to me? Who was she to decide my future? What did I do to deserve this?

Hidden in all these questions is the "why" that I described earlier, the search for an answer to reduce my suffering. However, plunging into this impossible quest was the very indication of my victimhood. By being angry and upset, I was giving this woman power she did not deserve.

When I finally recovered, I remember thinking "Take that, you bitch!" By proving her wrong, I believed I had set myself free from her victimization. But needing to prove yourself is yet another form of imprisonment. It stems from the primal human desire to feel seen and acknowledged, which is at the root of wanting to feel worthy and significant. However, as with all labels, the belief that you will internalize your desired state of "feeling worthy" through external validation is an illusion. Because nothing outside of you can truly define you, you become entrenched in a vicious cycle of trying to prove yourself to others. What freed me from this prison was forgiveness. You may wonder how you can forgive someone or something that is clearly wrong – *they hurt you!* True. But what will hurt you more is carrying their burden for the rest of your life. To forgive isn't to let someone off the hook; it's about setting yourself free. It's about letting go, which is an act of far greater power than holding on.

I have spent a lot of time pondering the reasons why healthcare professionals would say such awful things to their patients. My conclusion has always been: they're people too. They have their own ego that wants to feel significant. By viewing the patient as the problem, they are making the patient "wrong" while believing they are making themselves "right." The delivery of harsh prognoses provides that professional with a perceived escape from their own victimhood. After all, victimhood means feeling powerless against something you can't control. I'm no professional in the traditional sense of the word, but I can only imagine their inner voice would go something like this: *I'm a professional! I fix people! I should know how to help this person!* So when they feel they can't help, therefore threatening their professional identity, their ego will do everything possible to redeem itself. By labeling the patient as the incapable one, the incurable one, they have let themselves off the hook. In reality, all they've done is given up responsibility. Most of the time, when you say you "can't" do something, you're actually saying that you "won't" do it. Healthcare professionals do this by sending their patients off with discouraging labels, but you also do it by feeding your limiting beliefs.

30

TRIGGERS

Labeling something as a "trigger" is one of the most common manifestations of the victim role. It's a way of excusing yourself into powerlessness, for you cannot take action if you believe something outside of you is preventing you from doing so. *Seeing that skinny person triggered me, so now I cannot eat. My mom skipped breakfast, so now I am triggered to skip breakfast too. Someone on social media posted a triggering transformation photo that's made me relapse.* When you view each scenario objectively, you come to understand that the other person is completely unrelated to your actions. Does seeing a skinny person truly cause you to not be able to eat, or have you justified restriction by blaming an external circumstance? How does your mom's eating behavior have any influence on you putting food into your mouth? What gave the compilation of pixels on a screen the power to spiral you back into sickness? If another person's appearance or actions caused a specific result in another person, then everyone in the world would be walking around with an eating disorder.

To free yourself from a life of limitation means to stop giving external circumstances the power to drive your actions. The truth is that you will never be able to control what happens around you, but you can always control how you react to it. This takes work, especially in the beginning. By choosing to be a victim every time an unfavorable event occurred, you have conditioned your brain, and therefore created the habit, that experiencing a "trigger" will inevitably lead to an action that is not aligned with your core values. As long as you believe there's a cause-effect relationship between these "triggers" and your actions, there will be. What's triggering for one person is empowering for another, meaning your definition of triggering is highly subjective. Therefore, becoming trigger-proof starts with acknowledging this subjectivity and becoming aware of the situation as it is. What are the facts? Once you realize nothing outside of you has the power to change you, you create the most powerful change within yourself.

31

DIET CULTURE

The American writer and philosopher Elbert Hubbard said that "responsibility is the price of freedom." To elaborate on this, becoming free from limiting labels means taking responsibility for your actions. In a thin-obsessed, diet-culture-ridden society, this means developing a strong backbone and owning your truth. Freedom from diet culture isn't about *rejecting* diet culture, for what you resist persists. Freedom from diet culture and its labels – or any labels, for that matter – is about accepting your circumstances and choosing what to do in them.

You know that saying "If you don't prioritize your life, someone else will"? More appropriate would be "If you don't prioritize your life, a label will." For almost a decade, I attached infinite worth to countless labels, including healthy/unhealthy, normal, the number on the scale, body mass index, weight restored, and certain lifestyles/diets including vegetarian, vegan, whole-foods-plant-based, and clean eating. A massive part of the sway of diet culture is quite literally "influenced" by (online) public figures. You have Slim Kim talking about how lemon water and celery juice "cleanses her liver of toxins" while Jimmie Junkie claims that going to the gym is what "saved him from his eating disorder." More nuanced are the individuals who attribute their healed relationship with food to going "all in," or better said, any label that falls under the umbrella term "recovery." These "lifesaving labels" can be perceived almost as the flip side of victimhood. Rather than blaming their misery on a victimizer, they have attributed their so-called freedom to a so-called savior. Why so-called? Because nothing outside of you will save you. Anyone who bases their happiness and state of being on labels is not truly free. They toil to prove themselves, which might as well be slavery to another's opinion. So just as being "in recovery" isn't any better than having an eating disorder, being enslaved to whatever foundation you believe your happiness rests upon is equally incarcerating as believing yourself to be a victim.

32

GUILT

In contrast to the societal belief that guilt is a negative emotion, feeling guilty is a very important part of living a positive life. Similar to your identity, guilt is a direct reflection of who you believe you are. No baby is born feeling guilty for their fatness, a clear illustration of how fatphobia is simply a response to societal conditioning. The fears, insecurities, and occasional feelings of guilt arise through the development of your belief system, or the "code of conduct" that contains everything you've been conditioned to believe.

As a child, you are taught to say please and thank you when someone is generous or kind, that this is the "right" thing to do. You are also taught what is the "wrong" thing to do, such as lying or stealing. The more you act in alignment with what you have learned, and therefore have been conditioned to believe, the deeper these beliefs become cemented in your unique array of values.

What you value as "right" and "wrong" directly influences what you believe you "should" or "should not" do. You are told that you should say please and thank you because it's the "right" thing to do, just like you are told you should not steal or lie because it's the "wrong" thing to do. Where guilt fits into all of this is that it helps you course-correct. A universal truth about humanity is that everyone makes mistakes. I've stolen before, I've lied before, and I've done many things that caused me to feel guilty afterwards. Yet it's these feelings of guilt that taught me to not repeat the action that caused me to feel guilty in the first place.

You know what guilt feels like: it's a painful, gut-wrenching emotion that no one enjoys. But that's the very reason you experience it: so you avoid behaving in a way that leads to feeling guilty in the future. That being said, guilt is not a "bad" thing. It serves an important purpose, which is to inform you of how to act in a way that is aligned with your true values.

An eating disorder, or any external identity, twists your belief system to support its parasitic ego. When your actions rest on the beliefs of the parasite, you start behaving in a way that goes directly against your authentic values. Just like you are taught that you should or shouldn't act a certain way to make friends, or that saying please is right and stealing is wrong, diet culture tells you there are foods that you "should" and "shouldn't" eat and that certain foods are either "right" or "wrong."

Diet-cultural conditioning and your eating disorder go hand in hand, a relationship that can be understood through the metaphor of a viral infection. As you may know, a virus cannot reproduce alone; it must infect cells and use components of the host cell to replicate. Once a virus has established itself, it spreads through the body to produce systemic infection. In this metaphor, you are the host, your eating disorder is the virus, and diet culture is represented by the various passages that transport the virus throughout the body.

Similar to a virus that cannot multiply without a host cell, an eating disorder cannot exist without you. For this reason, it can be most helpful to use person-first language (person with an eating disorder) rather than identity-first language (disordered person) when referring to your illness. This semantic shift turns victimhood into ownership, for seeing the eating disorder as a separate entity gives you the power to slay the disease.

When a virus infects a host cell, it uses the cell's RNA to make copies of itself. As it infects the organism, it ends up destroying the possibility of its long-term survival in the process. In the same vein, your eating disorder hijacks all your unique qualities – persistence, strength, creativity – and turns them against you. To spread throughout an organism, a virus needs pathways that support its contamination. Depending on the virus, the bloodstream, lymphatic system, and gastrointestinal tract may be part of its breeding ground. Comparably, diet culture supports an eating disorder's manifestation through confirming its toxic beliefs. When your eating disorder believes honoring mental hunger is wrong and diet culture confirms this, you, as the host, suffer the consequences (in this case, increased mental hunger). However, because your survival instinct knows that honoring mental hunger is right – as it's what you need to do to live a life of abundance – you eventually give in and may suddenly find yourself staring into the bottom of an empty pint of ice cream.

Oh no! you think. I *shouldn't* have done that! This is so *wrong!* But is it really wrong? Who said you shouldn't have done that? The only reason you feel guilty after honoring your mental hunger is because your current belief system – one that's not your own – perceives honoring mental hunger as a sin. To course-correct, the metaphorical virus attempts to put you "back on track" through restriction and compensation. Of course, you now know that engaging in this restriction is the root cause of your suffering, which raises the question: How do you get rid of the guilt? You foster the growth of your authentic belief system.

33

DISCOVERY

"Don't you want to go back to who you were before your eating disorder?" was a common question throughout my years of eating disorder treatment. The truth was, I didn't. But more importantly, I couldn't. By the time I realized I was sick and tired of being sick and tired, I was an adult who wanted to live her life. Going back to who I was before my eating disorder would mean reverting to childhood, a naive state that my newfound awareness had far surpassed. Plus, if I were to be the same person I was before my eating disorder, I would get my eating disorder all over again! The realization that you will be a completely new person when you are recovered can be terrifying, as the lack of knowledge provides you with zero trust. It's this very uncertainty that led me to cling to the label of being "in recovery," as at least this gave me something familiar to hold on to. But as discussed previously, being in recovery is an illusion that prevents you from living a full life.

During a coaching session, a client and I were collectively pondering another word to replace recovery. Not because you need a label to house the complex journey of discovering your true self, but because labels coming from a place of love can provide next-level empowerment. We talked about how focusing on recovery keeps you stuck in it, prompting us to find the essence of being recovered from an eating disorder: discovery. Unlike "recovery," which is limiting and subjective, discovery opens you up to infinite possibilities. Unlike recovery, which most people don't want to start out of fear they'll "fail" at it, you cannot fail at discovery. Unlike recovery, which often feels like a losing game that's coated in the trepidation of doing it "wrong," discovery isn't about winning or losing. It's about finding out who you are.

Through discovery, I've found out that I'm autistic. I've learned that the words "healthy" and "normal" are subjective and that they act as one of the greatest barriers to overcoming extreme hunger. Through delving into the history of diagnoses and medical approaches, I've come to realize that the traditional healthcare system's views on weight and shape are fucked up beyond belief. Through discovery, I've welcomed the full potential of the unknown, which has paved a path of unimaginable abundance. I've internalized how simple reframes can make all the difference, one most relevant to this book being: is extreme hunger really a problem, or is it the solution to becoming free? Through discovery, I've learned that I enjoy food when I'm not eating "mindfully" and that there is inherently no "right" or "wrong" way to approach life. We are all unique humans with our own battles, our own victories, and our own stories. Now stop reading this one, and go live yours.

WHAT DID YOU THINK?

Thank you so much for reading my book! It would mean the world to me if you could take two minutes to leave a review on Amazon and Goodreads. Your words help other people find my words!

With love and gratitude,

Liv

ALSO BY LIVIA SARA

Rainbow Girl

Nourishing Neurodiversity

How to Get Out of Quasi Recovery

Be the first!

Join the Liv Label Free family and be the first to receive updates on Livia's latest books and content: www.livlabelfree.com/join

ENDNOTES

6. What Causes Extreme Hunger?

1. A.G. Dulloo, J. Jacquet, and L. Girardier, "Poststarvation Hyperphagia and Body Fat Overshooting in Humans: A Role for Feedback Signals from Lean and Fat Tissues," *American Journal of Clinical Nutrition* 65, no. 3 (1997): 717–723.

8. Physical Hunger

1. W.B. Cannon, "Organization for Physiological Homeostasis," *Physiological Reviews* 9, no. 3 (1929): 399–431.

12. Emotional Eating and Binge Eating

1. N.D. Berkman et al., "Management and Outcomes of Binge-Eating Disorder," *Comparative Effectiveness Reviews*, no. 160 (December 2015): Table 1.

17. Junk Food

1. R. Nickerson, "Confirmation Bias: A Ubiquitous Phenomenon in Many Guises," *Review of General Psychology* 2, no. 2 (June 1998): 175–220.

21. BMI

1. G. Eknoyan, "Adolphe Quetelet (1796–1874) – the Average Man and Indices of Obesity," *Nephrology Dialysis Transplantation* 23, no. 1 (January 2008): 47–51.

22. Weight Restoration and Redistribution

1. R.B. Harris, "Role of Set-Point Theory in Regulation of Body Weight," *FASEB Journal* 4, no. 15 (December 1990): 3310–3318.

23. The Nervous System

1. E. Mtui, G. Gruener, and P. Dockery, *Fitzgerald's Clinical Neuroanatomy and Neuroscience*, 8th ed. (Elsevier, 2020).
2. "What Are the Parts of the Nervous System?," NIH, Eunice Kennedy Shriver National Institute of Child Health and Human Development, rev. October 1, 2018.

3. C. Stangor and J. Walinga, "Putting It All Together: The Nervous System and the Endocrine System," in *Introduction to Psychology*, 1st Canadian ed. (B.C. Open Textbook Project, 2018).
4. J.N. Langley, The Autonomic Nervous System (W. Heffer & Sons, 1921).
5. S. Rosenberg, Accessing the Healing Power of the Vagus Nerve (North Atlantic Books, 2018).
6. S.W. Porges, The Polyvagal Theory: Neurophysiological Foundations of Emotions, Attachments, Communication, and Self-Regulation (W.W. Norton, 2011).
7. N. Habib, Activate Your Vagus Nerve: Unleash Your Body's Natural Ability to Heal (Ulysses Press, 2022).
8. K. Uvnäs-Moberg, "Gastrointestinal Hormones in Mother and Infant," *Acta Pædiatrica* 78 (1989): 88–93.
9. S.W. Porges, "The Polyvagal Perspective," *Biological Psychiatry* 74, no. 2 (February 2007): 116–143.
10. A.S. Caravaca, "Vagus Nerve Stimulation Promotes Resolution of Inflammation by a Mechanism That Involves Alox15 and Requires the α7nAChR Subunit," *PNAS* 119, no. 22: e2023285119.
11. C. Mercier, "Hughlings-Jackson on Evolution and Dissolution of the Nervous System," *Brain* 7, no. 2 (July 1884): 283–284.
12. B. Özdemir, C. Celik, and T. Oznur, "Assessment of Dissociation Among Combat-Exposed Soldiers with and without Posttraumatic Stress Disorder," *European Journal of Psychotraumatology* 6 (April 2015): 26657.
13. P.W. Andrews and J.A. Thomson Jr., "The Bright Side of Being Blue: Depression as an Adaptation for Analyzing Complex Problems," *Psychological Review* 116, no. 3 (July 2009): 620–654.

24. The Endocrine System

1. M. Dingman, Your Brain, Explained: What Neuroscience Reveals About Your Brain and Its Quirks (Nicholas Brealey, 2022).
2. D. Purves et al., eds., Neuroscience, 2nd ed. (Sinauer Associates, 2001), chapter 6.

25. Digestive Issues

1. K.S. Patel and A. Thavamani, "Physiology, Peristalsis," StatPearls, National Library of Medicine, rev. March 12, 2023.
2. A. Reddivari and P. Mehta, "Gastroparesis," StatPearls, National Library of Medicine, September 30, 2022.
3. D.M. Clarrett and C. Hachem, "Gastroesophageal Reflux Disease (GERD)," *Missouri Medicine* 115, no. 3 (2018): 214–218.
4. S.A. Janssen, A. Arntz, and S. Bouts, "Anxiety and Pain: Epinephrine-Induced Hyperalgesia and Attentional Influences," *Pain* 76, no. 3 (1998): 309–316.
5. I. Şimşek, "Irritable Bowel Syndrome and Other Functional Gastrointestinal Disorders," Supplement, *Journal of Clinical Gastroenterology* 45 (2011): S86–88.
6. M. Carabotti et al., "The Gut-Brain Axis: Interactions between Enteric Microbiota, Central and Enteric Nervous Systems," *Annals of Gastroenterology* 28, no. 2 (2015): 203–209.

7. M.L. Heiman and F.L. Greenway, "A Healthy Gastrointestinal Microbiome Is Dependent on Dietary Diversity," *Molecular Metabolism* 5, no. 5 (2016): 317–320; I. Bourdeau-Julien et al., "The Diet Rapidly and Differentially Affects the Gut Microbiota and Host Lipid Mediators in a Healthy Population," *Microbiome* 11 (2023); C. Xiao et al. "Associations of Dietary Diversity with the Gut Microbiome, Fecal Metabolites, and Host Metabolism: Results from 2 Prospective Chinese Cohorts," *American Journal of Clinical Nutrition* 116, no. 4 (2022): 1049–1058.
8. A.V. Kane, D.M. Dinh, and H.D. Ward, "Childhood Malnutrition and the Intestinal Microbiome," *Pediatric Research* 77 (2015): 256–262.
9. S. Magge and A. Lembo, "Low-FODMAP Diet for Treatment of Irritable Bowel Syndrome," *Gastroenterology and Hepatology* 8, no. 11 (2012): 739–745.
10. J. Chen, X. Chen, and C.H. Ho, "Recent Development of Probiotic Bifidobacteria for Treating Human Diseases," *Frontiers in Bioengineering and Biotechnology* 9 (2021): 770248; E. Dempsey and S.C. Corr, "Lactobacillus spp. for Gastrointestinal Health: Current and Future Perspectives," *Frontiers in Immunology* 13 (2022).
11. E.J. Baron, "Bilophila Wadsworthia: A Unique Gram-Negative Anaerobic Rod," *Anaerobe* 3, nos. 2–3 (1997): 83–86.
12. D. Vandeputte and M. Joossens, "Effects of Low and High FODMAP Diets on Human Gastrointestinal Microbiota Composition in Adults with Intestinal Diseases: A Systematic Review," *Microorganisms* 8, no. 11 (2020): 1638.
13. F. Musial, S. Klosterhalfen, and P. Enck, "Placebo Responses in Patients with Gastrointestinal Disorders," *World Journal of Gastroenterology* 13, no. 25 (2007): 3425–3429.
14. J.-H. Li et al., "[Unique Characteristics of "The Second Brain" – The Enteric Nervous System]," *Sheng Li Xue Bao* 72, no. 3 (2020): 382–390 [article in Chinese].
15. D. Purves et al., eds., "The Enteric Nervous System," in *Neuroscience*, 2nd ed. (Sinauer Associates, 2001).
16. N. Terry and K.G. Margolis, "Serotonergic Mechanisms Regulating the GI Tract: Experimental Evidence and Therapeutic Relevance," *Handbook of Experimental Pharmacology* 239 (2017): 319–342.
17. G. Eisenhofer et al., "Substantial Production of Dopamine in the Human Gastrointestinal Tract," *Journal of Clinical Endocrinology and Metabolism* 82, no. 11 (1997): 3864–3871.
18. V. Daugé et al., "A Probiotic Mixture Induces Anxiolytic- and Antidepressive-Like Effects in Fischer and Maternally Deprived Long Evans Rats," *Frontiers in Behavioral Neuroscience* 14 (2020).
19. R.M. Bin-Khattaf et al., "Probiotic Ameliorating Effects of Altered GABA/Glutamate Signaling in a Rodent Model of Autism," *Metabolites* 12, no. 8 (2022): 720.

26. Hormonal Changes

1. G.F. Allan et al., "Induction of the Progesterone Receptor Gene in Estrogen Target Cells Monitored by Branched DNA Signal Amplification," *Steroids* 66, no. 9 (2001): 663–671.
2. T.D. Müller et al., "Ghrelin," *Molecular Metabolism* 4, no. 6 (2015): 437–460.
3. D.E. Cummings and J. Overduin, "Gastrointestinal Regulation of Food Intake," *Journal of Clinical Investigation* 117, no. 1 (2007): 13–23.

4. H.A. Al-hussaniy, A.H. Alburghaif, and M.A. Naji, "Leptin Hormone and Its Effectiveness in Reproduction, Metabolism, Immunity, Diabetes, Hopes and Ambitions," *Journal of Medicine and Life* 14, no. 5 (2021): 600–605.
5. R.V. Considine et al., "Serum Immunoreactive-Leptin Concentrations In Normal-Weight and Obese Humans," *New England Journal of Medicine* 334, no. 5 (1996): 292–295.
6. J. Miyoung et al., "Leptin Rapidly Inhibits Hypothalamic Neuropeptide Y Secretion and Stimulates Corticotropin-Releasing Hormone Secretion in Adrenalectomized Mice," *Journal of Nutrition* 130, no. 11 (2000): 2813–2820.
7. V.A. Genchi et al., "Impaired Leptin Signalling in Obesity: Is Leptin a New Thermolipokine?," *International Journal of Molecular Sciences* 22, no. 12 (2021): 6445.
8. S. Guisinger, "Adapted to Flee Famine: Adding an Evolutionary Perspective on Anorexia Nervosa," *Psychological Review* 110, no. 4 (2003): 745–761.
9. A.M. Prentice, B.J. Hennig, and T. Fulford, "Evolutionary Origins of the Obesity Epidemic: Natural Selection of Thrifty Genes or Genetic Drift Following Predation Release?," *International Journal of Obesity* 32, no. 11 (2008): 1607–1610.
10. W.W. Gull, "V.—Anorexia Nervosa (Apepsia Hysterica, Anorexia Hysterica)," *Obesity Research* 5, no. 5 (1997): 387–510.
11. B. Otto et al., "Weight Gain Decreases Elevated Plasma Ghrelin Concentrations of Patients with Anorexia Nervosa," *European Journal of Endocrinology* 145, no. 5 (2001): 669–673; W.H. Kaye, "Neuropeptide Abnormalities in Anorexia Nervosa," *Psychiatry Research* 62, no. 1 (1996): 65–74; M. Méquinion et al., "Ghrelin: Central and Peripheral Implications in Anorexia Nervosa," *Frontiers in Endocrinology* 4 (2013); K.A. Gendall et al., "Leptin, Neuropeptide Y, and Peptide YY in Long-Term Recovered Eating Disorder Patients," *Biological Psychiatry* 46 (1999): 292–299.
12. American Psychiatric Association, "Other Specified Feeding or Eating Disorder," in Diagnostic and Statistical Manual of Mental Disorders, 5th ed. (APA, 2022), 353.
13. E. Kawasaki, "Type 1 Diabetes and Autoimmunity," *Clinical Pediatric Endocrinology* 23, no. 4 (2014): PMC4219937.
14. V. Baron and E. Van Obberghen, "[Mechanism of Insulin Action]," *Comptes Rendus des Seances de la Societe de Biologie et de ses Filiales* 189, no. 1 (1995): 25–41 [article in French].
15. B. Fletcher, M. Gulanick, and C. Lamendola, "Risk Factors for Type 2 Diabetes Mellitus," *Journal of Cardiovascular Nursing* 16, no. 2 (2002): 17–23.
16. J.F. Plows et al., "The Pathophysiology of Gestational Diabetes Mellitus," *International Journal of Molecular Sciences* 10, no. 11 (2018): 3342.
17. J.P. Kirwan et al., "Reversal of Insulin Resistance Postpartum Is Linked to Enhanced Skeletal Muscle Insulin Signaling," *Journal of Clinical Endocrinology & Metabolism* 89, no. 9 (2004): 4678–4684; A.D. Sonagra et al., "Normal Pregnancy-A State of Insulin Resistance," *Journal of Clinical & Diagnostic Research* 8, no. 11 (2014): CC01–CC03; M. Leoni et al., "Mechanisms of Insulin Resistance during Pregnancy," in *Evolving Concepts in Insulin Resistance*, ed. M. Infante (Intech Open, 2022).
18. A. Tsatsoulis et al., "Insulin Resistance: An Adaptive Mechanism Becomes Maladaptive in the Current Environment – An Evolutionary Perspective," *Metabolism* 62, no. 5 (2012): 622–633.
19. E. Shiloah et al., "Effect of Acute Psychotic Stress in Nondiabetic Subjects on Beta-Cell Function and Insulin Sensitivity," *Diabetes Care* 26, no. 5 (2003): 1462–

1467; F.G. Huffman et al., "The Association of Depression and Perceived Stress with Beta Cell Function between African and Haitian Americans with and without Type 2 Diabetes," *Journal of Diabetes Mellitus* 3, no. 4 (2013): 236–243; T. Parkulo, "The Effects of Chronic Stress and Exercise on Mouse Pancreatic Islet of Langerhans Morphology and Muscle Atrophy Gene Expression" (graduate thesis, West Virginia University, 2014); K. Bebbington et al., "203-OR: Characterizing Moment-to-Moment Fluctuations in Stress, Anxiety, and Blood Glucose Levels in Adolescents with Type 1 Diabetes," *Diabetes* 68, Supplement 1 (2019).
20. H. Yaribeygi et al., "Review Article: Molecular Mechanisms Linking Stress and Insulin Resistance,"*EXCLI Journal* 21 (2022): 317–334.
21. P.H. Black and L.D. Garbutt, "Stress, Inflammation and Cardiovascular Disease," *Journal of Psychosomatic Research* 52, no. 1 (2002): 1–23.
22. Tsatsoulis et al., "Insulin Resistance" (see note 18).
23. B.S. McEwen, "Protective and Damaging Effects of Stress Mediators," *New England Journal of Medicine* 338, no. 3 (1998): 171–179; E. Charmandari, C. Tsigos, and G. Chrousos, "Endocrinology of the Stress Response," *Annual Review of Physiology* 67 (2005): 259–284; A.J. Peckett, D.C. Wright, and M.C. Riddell, "The Effects of Glucocorticoids on Adipose Tissue Lipid Metabolism," *Metabolism* 60, no. 11 (2011): 1500–1510.
24. "Metabolism," Medline Plus Medical Encyclopedia, StatPearls, rev. July 21, 2022.
25. J. Hargrove, "Does the History of Food Energy Units Suggest a Solution to 'Calorie Confusion'?," *Nutrition Journal* 6 (2007): 44.
26. S. Sorrenti et al., "Iodine: Its Role in Thyroid Hormone Biosynthesis and Beyond," *Nutrients* 13, no. 12 (2021): 4469.
27. InformedHealth.org, "How Does the Thyroid Gland Work?," Institute for Quality and Efficiency in Health Care, rev. April 19, 2018.
28. L.S. Usdan, L. Khaodhiar, and C.M. Apovian, "The Endocrinopathies of Anorexia Nervosa," *Endocrine Practice* 14, no. 8 (2008): 1055–1063.
29. D.L. Mincer and I. Jialal, "Hashimoto Thyroiditis," StatPearls, National Library of Medicine, rev. July 29, 2023.
30. A. Clark et al., "Nutrition and Metabolism in Burn Patients," *Burns & Trauma* 5, no. 1 (2017): 11; J. Pravda, "Metabolic Theory of Septic Shock,"*World Journal of Critical Care Medicine* 3, no. 2 (2014): 45–54.
31. M.G. Jeschke, "Post-burn hypermetabolism: past, present and future," *Journal of Burn Care and Research* 37, no. 2 (2016): 86–96; M.G. Jeschke et al., "Long-Term Persistence of the Pathophysiologic Response to Severe Burn Injury," *PLoS One* 6, no. 7 (2011); e21245.
32. "Your Kidneys & How They Work," NIH, National Institute of Diabetes and Digestive and Kidney Diseases, rev. June 2018.
33. E.H. Larsen et al., "Osmoregulation and Excretion," *Comprehensive Physiology* 4, no. 2 (2014): 405–573.
34. B. Cuzzo, S.A. Padala, and S.L. Lappin, "Physiology, Vasopressin," StatPearls, National Library of Medicine, rev. August 14, 2023; J.H. Scott, M.A. Menouar, and R.J. Dunn, "Physiology, Aldosterone," StatPearls, National Library of Medicine, rev. May 1, 2023.
35. S. Rotenberg and J.J. McGrath, "Inter-Relation Between Autonomic and HPA Axis Activity in Children and Adolescents," *Biological Psychology* 117 (2016): 16–25.
36. D. Toufexis et al., "Stress and the Reproductive Axis," *Journal of Neuroendocrinology* 26, no. 9 (2014): 573–586.

37. A.Y. Herrera et al., "Estradiol Therapy After Menopause Mitigates Effects of Stress on Cortisol and Working Memory," *Journal of Clinical Endocrinology & Metabolism* 102, no. 12 (2017): 4457–4466; D.R. Rubinow et al., "Testosterone Suppression of CRH-Stimulated Cortisol in Men," Neuropsychopharmacology 30, no. 10 (2005): 1906–1912.
38. C.L. Shufelt, T. Torbati, and E. Dutra, "Hypothalamic Amenorrhea and the Long-Term Health Consequences," *Seminars in Reproductive Medicine* 35, no. 3 (2017): 256–262.
39. M.L. Elsaie, "Hormonal Treatment of Acne Vulgaris: An Update," *Clinical, Cosmetic and Investigational Dermatology* 9 (2016): 241–248.
40. W. Wharton et al., "Neurobiological Underpinnings of the Estrogen–Mood Relationship," *Current Psychiatry Reviews* 8, no. 3 (2012): 247–256.
41. D. Dfarhud, M. Malmir, and M. Khanahmadi, "Happiness & Health: The Biological Factors – Systematic Review Article," *Iran Journal of Public Health* 43, no. 11 (2014): 1468–1477.
42. Wharton et al., "Neurobiological Underpinnings of the Estrogen–Mood Relationship" (see note 40).
43. R. Hardy and D. Kuh, "Change in Psychological and Vasomotor Symptom Reporting during the Menopause," *Social Science & Medicine* 55, no. 11 (2002): 1975–1988; N.F. Woods, A. Mariella, and E.S. Mitchell, "Patterns of Depressed Mood Across the Menopausal Transition: Approaches to Studying Patterns in Longitudinal Data," *Acta Obstetricia et Gynecologica Scandinavica* 81, no. 7 (2002): 623–632; P.R. Albert, F. Vahid-Ansari, and C. Luckhart, "Serotonin-Prefrontal Cortical Circuitry in Anxiety and Depression Phenotypes: Pivotal Role of Pre- and Post-Synaptic 5-HT1A Receptor Expression," *Frontiers in Behavioral Neuroscience* 6, no. 8 (2014): 199; C.M. Portas, B. Bjorvatn, and R. Ursin, "Serotonin and the Sleep/Wake Cycle: Special Emphasis on Microdialysis Studies," *Progress in Neurobiology* 60, no. 1 (2000): 13–35; J. Lee et al., "Sleep Disorders and Menopause," *Journal of Menopausal Medicine* 25, no. 2 (2019): 83–87.
44. L.A. Rybaczyk et al., "An Overlooked Connection: Serotonergic Mediation of Estrogen-Related Physiology and Pathology," *BMC Women's Health* 5 (2005): 12.
45. A. Bartels and S. Zeki, "The Neural Correlates of Maternal and Romantic Love," *NeuroImage* 21, no. 3 (2004): 1155–1166; J.B. Nitschke et al., "Orbitofrontal Cortex Tracks Positive Mood in Mothers Viewing Pictures of Their Newborn Infants," *NeuroImage* 21, no. 2 (2004): 583–592; L. Strathearn et al., "What's in a Smile? Maternal Brain Responses to Infant Facial Cues,"*Pediatrics* 122, no. 1 (2008): 40–51.
46. H.K. Laurent and J.C. Ablow, "A Face a Mother Could Love: Depression-Related Maternal Neural Responses to Infant Emotion Faces,"*Social Neuroscience* 8, no. 3 (2013): 228–239.
47. American Psychiatric Association, "Premenstrual Dysphoric Disorder," in Diagnostic and Statistical Manual of Mental Disorders, 5th ed. (APA, 2022), 171.
48. C.A. Wilson, C.W. Turner, and W.R. Keye Jr., "Firstborn Adolescent Daughters and Mothers with and without Premenstrual Syndrome: A Comparison," *Journal of Adolescent Health* 12, no. 2 (1991): 130–137; K.S. Kendler et al., "Genetic and Environmental Factors in the Aetiology of Menstrual, Premenstrual and Neurotic Symptoms: A Population-Based Twin Study," *Psychological Medicine* 22, no. 1 (February 1992): 85–100; J.T. Condon, "The Premenstrual Syndrome: A Twin Study," *British Journal of Psychology* 162 (April 1993): 481–486; K.S. Kendler et al.,

"Longitudinal Population-Based Twin Study of Retrospectively Reported Premenstrual Symptoms and Lifetime Major Depression," *American Journal of Psychology* 155, no. 9 (September 1998): 1234–1240.

49. L. Huo et al., "Risk for Premenstrual Dysphoric Disorder Is Associated with Genetic Variation in ESR1, the Estrogen Receptor Alpha Gene," *Biological Psychiatry* 62, no. 8 (October 2007): 925–933; V. Dhingra et al., Serotonin Receptor 1A C(-1019)G Polymorphism Associated With Premenstrual Dysphoric Disorder," *Obstetric Gynecology* 110, no. 4 (October 2007): 788–792.

50. E.R. Raffi and M.P. Freeman, "The Etiology of Premenstrual Dysphoric Disorder: 5 Interwoven Pieces," *Current Psychiatry* 16, no. 9 (2017): 21–28.

51. M. Gao et al., "Global and Regional Prevalence and Burden for Premenstrual Syndrome and Premenstrual Dysphoric Disorder," *Medicine* (Baltimore) 101, no. 1 (2022): e28528.

52. H. Obaydi and B.K. Puri, "Prevalence of Premenstrual Syndrome in Autism: A Prospective Observer-Rated Study," *Journal of International Medical Research* 36, no. 2 (2008): 268–272.

53. F. Dorani et al., "Prevalence of Hormone-Related Mood Disorder Symptoms in Women with ADHD," *Journal of Psychiatric Research* 133 (2021): 10–15.

54. B. Chakrabarti et al., "Genes Related to Sex Steroids, Neural Growth, and Social-Emotional Behavior Are Associated with Autistic Traits, Empathy, and Asperger Syndrome," *Autism Research* 2, no. 3 (2009): 157–177; J. Veenstra-VanderWeele et al., "Autism Gene Variant Causes Hyperserotonemia, Serotonin Receptor Hypersensitivity, Social Impairment and Repetitive Behavior," *Proceedings of the National Academy of Sciences of the United States of America* 109, no. 14 (2012): 5469–5474.

55. S.-H. Shim et al., "A Case-Control Association Study of Serotonin 1A Receptor Gene and Tryptophan Hydroxylase 2 Gene in Attention Deficit Hyperactivity Disorder," *Progress in Neuro-Psychopharmacology and Biological Psychiatry* 34, no. 6 (2010): 974–979.

56. M. Andersson et al., "Serotonin Transporter Availability in Adults with Autism—A Positron Emission Tomography Study," *Molecular Psychiatry* 26 (2021): 1647–1658; K. Nakamura et al., "Brain Serotonin and Dopamine Transporter Bindings in Adults with High-Functioning Autism," *Archives of General Psychiatry* 67, no. 1 (2010): 59–68; C.L. Muller, A.M.J. Anacker, and J. Veenstra-VanderWeele, "The Serotonin System in Autism Spectrum Disorder: From Biomarker to Animal Models," *Neuroscience* 321 (2016): 24–41.

57. E. Banerjee and K. Nandagopal, "Does Serotonin Deficit Mediate Susceptibility to ADHD?," *Neurochemistry International* 82 (2015): 52–68; J.F. Quist et al., "The Serotonin 5-HT1B Receptor Gene and Attention Deficit Hyperactivity Disorder | Molecular Psychiatry," *Molecular Psychiatry* 8 (2003): 98–102.

58. N. Dubey et al., "The ESC/E(Z) Complex, an Effector of Response to Ovarian Steroids, Manifests an Intrinsic Difference in Cells from Women with Premenstrual Dysphoric Disorder," *Molecular Psychiatry* 22, no. 8 (2017): 1172–1184.

59. Raffi and Freeman, "The Etiology of Premenstrual Dysphoric Disorder" (see note 50); E.G. Spratt et al., "Enhanced Cortisol Response to Stress in Children in Autism," *Journal of Autism and Developmental Disorders* 42, no. 1 (2011): 75–81; G. Makris et al., "Stress System Activation in Children and Adolescents with Autism Spectrum Disorder," *Frontiers in Neuroscience* 15 (2021); C. Sharpley et al., "Further Evidence of HPA-Axis Dysregulation and Its Correlation with Depression in

Autism Spectrum Disorders: Data from Girls," *Physiology and Behavior* 167 (2016): 110–117.

60. J. Arendt and A. Aulinas, "Physiology of the Pineal Gland and Melatonin," in *Endotext*, ed. K.R. Feingold et al. (MDText.com, 2000); R.Y. Moore, "Suprachiasmatic Nucleus," in *International Encyclopedia of the Social & Behavioral Sciences*, ed. N.J. Smelser and P.B. Baltes (Pergamon, 2001), 15290–15294.

61. B.H. Lee, B. Hille, and D.-S. Koh, "Serotonin Modulates Melatonin Synthesis as an Autocrine Neurotransmitter in the Pineal Gland," *PNAS* 118, no. 43 (2021): e2113852118.

62. D.M. Richard et al., "L-Tryptophan: Basic Metabolic Functions, Behavioral Research and Therapeutic Indications," *International Journal of Tryptophan Research* 2 (2009): 45–60.

ABOUT THE AUTHOR

Livia Sara is an autism advocate and eating disorder survivor that now helps others overcome their own mental barriers through her courses and coaching programs. She is the author of the blog livlabelfree.com and the host of the Liv Label Free Podcast. Livia is a lifelong learner that loves listening to audiobooks, going on walks, and reading the latest science on all things neurodiversity and eating disorders!

youtube.com/@LivLabelFree
instagram.com/livlabelfree
facebook.com/livlabelfree

www.ingramcontent.com/pod-product-compliance
Lightning Source LLC
Chambersburg PA
CBHW050108170426
43198CB00014B/2503